Seizure Freedom: Clinical, Research and Quality of Life Perspectives

Edited by

MICHAEL R. TRIMBLE

Professor of Behavioural Neurology, Institute of Neurology and
Consultant Physician in Psychological Medicine,
National Hospitals for Neurology and Neurosurgery, London, UK

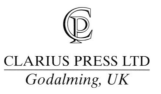

CLARIUS PRESS LTD
Godalming, UK

Published by

Clarius Press Ltd
135 Peperharow Road, Godalming,
Surrey GU7 2PW, UK

British Library Cataloguing in Publication Data
A catalogue record for this book is available from the British Library

ISBN 978-0-9542279-6-8

Composition by Wellset Repro Ltd, Cranleigh, Surrey, UK
Printed and bound in Great Britain by Biddles Ltd, King's Lynn

Contents

Contributors

Richard Appleton, The Roald Dahl EEG Unit, Department of Neurology, Royal Liverpool Children's NHS Trust (Alder Hey), Eaton Road, Liverpool L12 2AP, UK

Gus A. Baker, Division of Neurosciences, Clinical Science Centre for Research and Education, University of Liverpool, Lower Lane, Fazakerley, Liverpool L9 7LJ, UK

Ettore Beghi, Department of Neurology, Istituto di Ricerche Farmacologiche 'Mario Negri', Milano, Italy

Massimiliano Beghi, Department of Psychiatry, University of Milano-Bicocca, Ospedale 'San Gerardo', Monza, Italy

David A. Bell, Victor Horsley department of Neurosurgery, The National Hospital for Neurology and Neurosurgery and Institute of Neurology, Queen Square, London WC1N 3BG, UK

Norman Delanty, Department of Clinical Neurological Science, Royal College of Surgeons in Ireland, Beaumont Hospital, Dublin 9, Ireland

Carl B. Dodrill, Regional Epilepsy Center (Box 359745), Harborview Medical Center, 325 Ninth Avenue, Seattle, WA 98104-2499, USA

Jerome Engel, Department of Neurology, David Geffen School of Medicine at UCLA, 710 Westwood Plaza, Suite 1-250, Los Angeles, CA 90095-1769, USA

Ann Jacoby, Division of Public Health, 3rd Floor Wheelan Building, The Quadrangle, Brownlow Hill, Liverpool L69 3GP, UK

Peter Kinirons, Department of Clinical Neurological Science, Royal College of Surgeons in Ireland, Beaumont Hospital, Dublin 9, Ireland

Andrew M. McEvoy, Victor Horsley department of Neurosurgery, The National Hospital for Neurology and Neurosurgery and Institute of Neurology, Queen Square, London WC1N 3BG, UK

Lina Nashef, King's College Hospital, Denmark Hill, London SE5 9RS, UK

Asla Pitkänen, A.I. Virtanen Institute for Molecular Sciences, Department of Neurobiology, University of Kuopio, PO Box 1627 (street address: Neulaniementie 2) FIN-70 211 Kuopio, Finland

Matti Sillanpää, Departments of Child Neurology and Public Health, University of Turku, Turku, Finland

Susan C. Usiskin, The National Hospital for Neurology and Neurosurgery, Queen Square, London WC1N 3BG, UK

Matthew C. Walker, Department of Clinical and Experimental Epilepsy, Institute of Neurology, UCL, London WC1N 3BG, UK

Preface

It is now widely acknowledged that the majority of patients who develop seizures and who have a diagnosis of epilepsy will go into remission. This may occur spontaneously, but figures of about 50-65% of patients who are treated with anti-epileptic drugs becoming seizure-free seem to be accepted. Obviously to achieve seizure freedom depends upon many factors, some of which are biological and related to the epilepsy, others of which are sociological and related to the patient and their family and carers. However, until recently it was the case that the remainder of patients would continue to have seizures, at various frequencies, and a hardcore of patients, perhaps 20-30% would become intractable to medications.

The main aim of managing epilepsy must be to achieve seizure freedom, although not if this can only be achieved at great burden to the patient. In the past 20 years or so, treatments to achieve a greater percentage of people becoming seizure-free have been developed. These include an array of new anti-epileptic drugs, surgical interventions such as temporal lobectomy, but with now a much more sophisticated pre-operative workup than had been possible previously, and alternatives such as vagus nerve stimulation.

There are numerous texts on epilepsy and its management, most of them dealing in a very scientific or pragmatic way with epilepsy and its complications, but in this monograph the editor has been concerned with the difficult subject of seizure freedom. To these ends the book attempts to summarise what it is that may identify patients who fail to become seizure-free, what therapeutic strategies there may be to increase the number of patients who become seizure-free, and also to examine the effects of seizure freedom on psychosocial variables such as quality of life.

The chapters begin with an attempt to understand which populations become seizure-free, and epidemiological surveys which allow some degree of initial prediction are reviewed. The second chapter is concerned with the issue of neuroprotection; is it possible not only to inhibit seizures, but also to interfere with the possible progressive underlying processes of the epilepsy, and how might anti-epileptic drugs be related to that?

In order for medications to be effective, seizures have to be turned off. The underlying mechanisms that may relate to this, being central to their mode of action, are the subject of the third chapter.

There then follows four chapters related to treatment, which include the use of anti-epileptic drugs, surgical options, and a chapter dealing with the management of children with epilepsy. The other chapter examines some possible reasons for treatment resistance, reviewing the underlying potential pharmacokinetic, pharmacodynamic and biochemical factors that may be of relevance.

The final chapters of the book look at the benefits of seizure frequency from a patient's point of view, and the effects of seizures and seizure freedom on cognition, driving, and quality of life.

It is hoped that this book will provide a further impetus to study the brain mechanisms which may lead to seizure freedom, and give clinicians looking after people with epilepsy some fresh insights perhaps into management of the disorder. It will hopefully open up some new ideas which might lead to further research helping future generations of patients with epilepsy achieve the ultimate goal, namely seizure freedom.

MICHAEL R. TRIMBLE
London
July 2006

1

Epidemiology:
Which Patient Populations become
Seizure-Free

MATTI SILLANPÄÄ

*Departments of Child Neurology and Public Health,
University of Turku, Turku, Finland*

INTRODUCTION

Seizure freedom is the most desirable target in the management of epilepsy, wanted by the patient, relatives, health care workers and society in general. Understandably, among the first questions asked by the patient or their relatives after the onset of epilepsy is that about their future with regard to seizure occurrence. It is in many ways impossible to give an answer to the question regarding individual prognosis, because so many factors may affect the outcome. "It is tough to make predictions—particularly about the future", a Spanish proverb from the 17th century says it all! Recent outcome prediction models have been proved incorrect in predicting the outcome of childhood epilepsy in about one third of the patients (Geelhoed *et al.*, 2005) and at best, probabilities based on population studies can only be given. Probabilities derived from studies based on unbiased cohorts may substantially help patients understand their real chances of seizure freedom, and in any case, the treating doctor's role is to maintain the hope of favourable outcome and encourage the patient to aim to that end.

SEIZURE FREEDOM AFTER FIRST UNPROVOKED SEIZURE

Estimates of overall chances of seizure freedom after a first attack vary widely, from 20% to 70% (Hauser *et al.*, 1982; Annegers *et al.*, 1986; Elwes *et al.*, 1984), depending on the study design. In their meta-analysis of 16 reports,

Berg and Shinnar (1991) suggested that seizure freedom was an average of 51%. The chances of such a good outcome were largely explained by three methodological factors: whether the patients were recruited after a first seizure or after several seizures; time directionality; and the interval between the first seizure and the first medical assessment.

The chance of remaining seizure-free decreases with an increasing number of follow-up years, from 84% after one year to 79% after two years, to 73% after three years, and 66% after five years from the first seizure (Hauser et al., 1982; 1990). In childhood, the chances of seizure freedom are of similar magnitude and order, from 40% to 75% up to seven years of age (Pearce and Mackintosh, 1979; Hirtz et al., 1984; Camfield et al., 1985a). The studies do not reveal therefore any differences in the chances of seizure freedom between children and adults.

In the study of Shinnar and colleagues (1990), after a three-year follow-up from a first seizure, 74% of children with a normal neurological development but only 60% of children with abnormal development were still seizure-free. Other factors have also been examined. Age at onset of less than two years (Hirtz et al., 1984) or more than 50 years (Hopkins et al., 1988) has been suggested to favour seizure freedom. A normal EEG as opposed to one with abnormalities argues for a good outcome in both children (Shinnar et al., 1990) and adults (Hopkins et al., 1988) particularly if the neurological status is normal (Annegers et al., 1986; Hopkins et al., 1988; Hauser et al., 1990; Shinnar et al., 1990; Camfield et al., 1985a), the aetiology is idiopathic and seizures are primarily generalised (Annegers et al., 1986; Hirtz et al., 1984; Shinnar et al., 1990). Remarkably, an idiopathic status epilepticus of half an hour duration, whether convulsive or non-convulsive, does not appear to affect seizure outcome (Hauser et al., 1990; Shinnar et al., 1990).

Anti-epileptic drug therapy may improve the outcome in newly diagnosed patients, but the effect is not necessarily successful. Despite a good treatment compliance, only 59% of 82 children were seizure-free in a Canadian study (Camfield et al., 1985b). In another study, one hundred patients, consecutively hospitalised for epilepsy, were randomised to take either vigabatrin or carbamazepine treatment. At one year follow-up, 65% of carbamazepine-treated and 52% of vigabatrin-treated were in remission (Kälviäinen, 1992). It is intriguing to note that in yet another, population-based cohort from the same geographic area, 52% of 33 completely AED-untreated patients with epilepsy were in terminal remission of two years or more after 20-year follow-up! (Keränen, 1988).

SEIZURE FREEDOM IN EPILEPSIES

Various definitions of seizure freedom or remission have been applied in the literature ranging from six months to 10 years. According to the recommendation of the ILAE Commission 1997, seizure freedom of five years or more means that the epilepsy is no longer "active" and, vice versa, five or more years from the last seizure means five-year seizure freedom. Accordingly, at least a five-year follow-up is needed to arrive at a five-year terminal remission. A shorter-term remission may also be applied, keeping in mind an often used definition of drug resistance namely if seizure freedom is not achieved within one to three years using at least two appropriate drugs in an adequate way. If the seizure freedom is not achieved within that time, it is less likely to be attained later (Kwan and Brodie, 2000; Arts et al., 1999).

In some studies of the self-reports of patients with epilepsy, in terms of quality of life, being in remission or having seizures are not so important as being off medication, i.e. they feel medication can be even more disturbing than seizures (Sillanpää et al., 2004). Accordingly, seizure freedom off medication is the goal to be sought after by the patients. In a very long-term follow-up investigation, about half the patients who were seizure-free were also without medication (Annegers et al., 1979; Sillanpää et al., 1998).

Few prospective long-term follow-up studies based on population-cohorts exist on people with epilepsy (Annegers et al., 1979; Brorson and Wranne, 1987; Cockerell et al., 1995; Sillanpää et al., 1998). Complementary information is available from some longitudinal institution-based reports (Okuma and Kumashiro, 1981; Oka et al., 1989; Sofijanov, 1982). Approximately two thirds of patients will achieve terminal seizure freedom of five years or more. In contrast to the studies after the first unprovoked seizure already quoted, the longer the follow-up is in population-based studies, the better are the chances for seizure freedom (Sillanpää, 2000; Annegers et al., 1979; Sofijanov, 1982). At least one five-year period of seizure remission—that need not mean absence of later relapses—is achieved during long-term follow-up by 80% of patients with newly diagnosed childhood onset epilepsy (Annegers et al., 1979; Sillanpää and Schmidt, 2006). About half the patients will achieve an early remission (during 12 months from onset of therapy) (Sillanpää and Schmidt, 2006; Annegers et al., 1979; Arts et al., 2004).

The use of the ILAE classification of epilepsies and epileptic syndromes (1989), or any other classification, shows that epilepsies are heterogeneous both by phenomenology, aetiology and in response to anti-epileptic pharmacotherapy (Semah, 2005). The prognosis is good to excellent in benign types of localisation related epilepsy (including benign rolandic, frontal and occipital epilepsies), childhood absence epilepsy, benign myoclonic epilepsy of infancy, and generalised tonic-clonic epilepsy occurring on awakening or independently of the sleep-wake cycle as described by Janz (1969). These epilepsies are either self-limiting or easily controlled with medication.

Localisation related epilepsies are less amenable to drug treatment, may benefit from surgery, or may prove to be completely intractable. A virtually complete intractability is mostly found in patients with a cerebral deficit of congenital origin. They include lesional, developmental, chromosomal and metabolic conditions that are often progressive by nature (Sillanpää, 2005).

PREDICTORS OF ACHIEVING SEIZURE FREEDOM

In pairwise comparisons, an abundance of individual factors has emerged which have been presented as significant predictors of seizure outcome. However, many of the individual factors are inter-dependent and may interact with each other. Independent predictors derived from multivariate analyses are of much more importance in clinical work. The predictors of successful outcome can be classified into three categories: low initial susceptibility to seizures, normal brain structures, and a good early effect of drug therapy (Table 1).

Although there is no consensus in the literature about factors which reliably predict seizure outcome, the following phenomenology and course of events may characterise a patient who has epilepsy of good prognosis. An intellectually and neurologically normal patient who has had no neonatal seizures and who has had only a few unprovoked seizures of one (not complex partial) type, of genetic or unknown origin after intensive neuroimaging studies, and in whom adequate initial medication gives a good early response.

Age at onset of epilepsy in childhood is one of the most controversial issues as seen in Table 1. No distinct age which is predictive of future seizure freedom can be assumed. Taking all ages, at 10 years after diagnosis, a five-year seizure freedom off medication has been seen in patients with diagnoses at less than 10 years, 10 to 19 years, 20 to 59 years, and 60 years and over in 51%, 40%, 28%, and 6%, respectively (Annegers et al., 1979).

PERMANENCE OF SEIZURE FREEDOM

Patients with newly diagnosed epilepsy and at least one five-year remission, in long-term follow-up, will be more likely to survive than those who never ex-perience such a remission (91% vs 45%, p<0.0001) (Sillanpää, to be published). Of the survivors, the risk of at least one relapse is 14-33% (Sillanpää and Schmidt, 2006; Arts et al., 2004; Annegers et al., 1979). The risk is some-what higher among the late relapsers than the early relapsers (57% vs 49%).

Table 1. Reported significant predictors of long-term good outcome of epilepsy in univariate and multivariate analyses

Predictor	References* Significant association in univariate analysis	Independent predictor in multivariate analysis
Low initial susceptibility to seizures		
–No previous neonatal seizures	1	1
–Age at onset <144 mo vs. ≥144 mo	1	
–Age at onset ≤12 mo		1
–Age at onset 12-144 mo vs. <12 mo		1
–Age at onset 12-88 mo vs. <12 mo or >88 mo	3	
–Age at onset 24-36 mo vs. other ages <16 yrs	6	
–Low number of seizures before medication	1,2,3,5,7	2
–1 or 2 seizures before medication		1
–<1 seizure/mo before medication	2	2
–Duration of seizure disorder ≤12 mo	6	
–Low number of seizures during first 6 mo before medication	1	
–Low number of seizures 6 mo after presentation	8	
–Low number of seizures during second 6 mo before medication	1	
–Number of seizures 0 to 1 between 6 and 12 mo with medication		1
–One seizure type only	6	
–Absence of complex partial seizures	4	4
–Seizures in wakefulness only	2,3	
–Occurrence of status epilepticus	2	2
–Postictal signs	7	7
–Normal vs. abnormal EEG	1	
–Normal vs. "epileptiform" EEG	7	
–Normal vs. abnormal background in EEG	1	
–No severely abnormal background activity	3	
Normal brain structures		
–Genetic or unknown vs. known etiology	1,2,3,5,6	2
–Genetic or unknown, and no febrile seizures		7
–Normal vs. abnormal neurological development	3	
–Normal vs. abnormal neurological status	1,2,3	
–Normal intelligence vs. retardation	1	1
–No personality disturbances	3	
–No psychotic disturbance	3	
–No partial symptomatic seizures	7	
Good drug effect		
–Good vs. poor early effect	2	2
–Good vs. poor effect with first drug	5	

* 1 = Camfield *et al.*, 1993. 2 = Sillanpää., 1993. 3 = Okuma and Kumashiro, 1981. 4 = Sillanpää *et al.*, 1998.
5 = Kwan and Brodie, 2000. 6 = Sofijanov, 1982; Beghi and Tognoni, 1988. 7 = Arts *et al.*, 2004.
8 = MacDonald *et al.*, 2000.

On a very long-term follow-up, both the early and late remitters will achieve approximately the same terminal seizure freedom rate of at least five years (82% vs 83%) (Sillanpää and Schmidt, 2006).

CONCLUSIONS

Anti-epileptic drug treatment is the most important strategy to prevent re-occurrence of seizures and make the patient seizure-free. Seizure freedom is, however, only part of total care and quality of life of the patient with epilepsy. Seizure freedom is likely to be best achieved in patients who have no brain structural pathology, whose seizures are few before initiation of therapy and whose seizures are abolished totally within a few months from the onset of an adequate therapy. The responsibility for the effectiveness of the treatment is shared by the treating doctor, the patient, and people in daily and close proximity to the patient who can best help in maintaining therapeutic optimism.

REFERENCES

Annegers, J. F., Hauser, W. A. and Elveback, L. R. (1979). Remission of seizures and relapse in patients with epilepsy. *Epilepsia, 20,* 729-737.

Annegers, J. F., Shirts, S. B., Hauser, W. A. and Kurland, L. T. (1986). Risk of recurrence after an initial unprovoked seizure. *Epilepsia, 27,* 43-50.

Arts, W. F., Geerts, A. T., Brouwer, O. F., Boudewyn Peters, A. C., Stroink, H. and van Donselaar, C. A. (1999). The early prognosis of epilepsy in childhood: the prediction of a poor outcome. The Dutch study of epilepsy in childhood. *Epilepsia, 40,* 726-734.

Arts, W. F., Brouwer, O. F., Peters, A. C., Stroink, H., Peeters, E. A., Schmitz, P. I., van Donselaar, C. A. and Geerts, A. T. (2004). Course and prognosis of childhood epilepsy: 5-year follow-up of the Dutch study of epilepsy in childhood. *Brain, 127,* 1774-1784.

Beghi, E. and Tognoni, G. (1988). Prognosis of epilepsy in newly referred patients: a multicenter prospective study. Collaborative Group for the Study of Epilepsy. *Epilepsia, 29,* 236-243.

Berg, A. T. and Shinnar, S. (1991). The risk of seizure recurrence following a first unprovoked seizure: a quantitative review. *Neurology, 41,* 965-972.

Brorson, L. O. and Wranne, L. (1987). Long-term prognosis in childhood epilepsy: survival and seizure prognosis. *Epilepsia, 28,* 324-330.

Camfield, P. R., Camfield, C. S., Dooley, J. M., Tibbles, J. A., Fung, T. and Garner, B. (1985a). Epilepsy after a first unprovoked seizure in childhood. *Neurology, 35,* 1657-1660.

Camfield, P. R., Camfield, C. S., Smith, E. C. and Tibbles, J. A. (1985b). Newly treated childhood epilepsy: a prospective study of recurrences and side effects. *Neurology, 35,* 722-725.

Camfield, C., Camfield, P., Gordon, K., Smith, B. and Dooley, J. (1993). Outcome of childhood epilepsy: a population-based study with a simple predictive scoring system for those treated with medication. Epilepsy after a first unprovoked seizure in childhood. *J Pediatr, 122,* 861-868.

Cockerell, O. C., Johnson, A. L., Sander, J. W., Hart, Y. M. and Shorvon, S. D. (1995). Remission of epilepsy: results from the National General Practice Study of Epilepsy. *Lancet, 346,* 140-144.

Elwes, R. D., Johnson, A. L., Shorvon, S. D. and Reynolds, E. H. (1984). The prognosis for seizure control in newly diagnosed epilepsy. *N Engl J Med, 311,* 944-947.

Geelhoed, M., Boerrigter, A. O., Camfield, P., Geerts, A. T., Arts, W., Smith, B. and Camfield, C. (2005). The accuracy of outcome prediction models for childhood-onset epilepsy. *Epilepsia, 46,* 1526-1532.

Hauser, W. A., Anderson, V. E., Loewenson, R. B. and McRoberts, S. M. (1982). Seizure recurrence after a first unprovoked seizure. *N Engl J Med, 307,* 522-528.

Hauser, W. A., Rich, S. S., Annegers, J. F. and Anderson, V. E. (1990). Seizure recurrence after a 1st unprovoked seizure: an extended follow-up. *Neurology, 40,* 1163-1170.

Hirtz, D. G., Ellenberg, J. H. and Nelson, K. B. (1984). The risk of recurrence of nonfebrile seizures in children. *Neurology, 34,* 637-641.

Hopkins, A., Garman, A. and Clarke, C. (1988). The first seizure in adult life. Value of clinical features, electroencephalography, and computerised tomographic scanning in prediction of seizure recurrence. *Lancet, 1,* 721-726.

Janz, D. (1969, p. 456.) *Die Epilepsien,* Thieme, Stuttgart.

Kälviäinen, R. (1992) *Newly diagnosed epileptic seizure disorder in adults. A prospective follow-up study on 100 patients.* Doctoral Thesis. Department of Neuroscience & Neurology, University of Kuopio, No. 24.

Keränen, T. (1988). *Epilepsy in adults. An epidemiological study in eastern Finland.*, University of Kuopio. Department of Neurology. Series of Reports No. 10, p. 43., Kuopio.

Kwan, P. and Brodie, M. J. (2000). Early identification of refractory epilepsy. *N Engl J Med,* **342,** 314-319.

MacDonald, B. K., Johnson, A. L., Goodridge, D. M., Cockerell, O. C., Sander, J. W. and Shorvon, S. D. (2000). Factors predicting prognosis of epilepsy after presentation with seizures. *Ann Neurol,* **48,** 833-841.

Oka, E., Yamatogi, Y., Ohtsuka, Y. and Ohtahara, S. (1989). Clinical course and prognosis of childhood epilepsy. *Acta Paediatr Jpn,* **31,** 259-266.

Okuma, T. and Kumashiro, H. (1981). Natural history and prognosis of epilepsy: report of a multi-institutional study in Japan. The group for the study of prognosis of epilepsy in Japan. *Epilepsia,* **22,** 35-53.

Pearce, J. L. and Mackintosh, H. T. (1979). Prospective study of convulsions in childhood. *N Z Med J,* **89,** 1-3.

Semah, F. (2005). Definition of intractability is a function of epilepsy syndrome. In: Miller, J.W. and Silbergeld, D.L. (Eds), *Epilepsy Surgery: Principles and Controversies.* Taylor & Francis, New York, pp. 20-25.

Shinnar, S., Berg, A. T., Moshe, S. L., Petix, M., Maytal, J., Kang, H., Goldensohn, E. S. and Hauser, W. A. (1990). Risk of seizure recurrence following a first unprovoked seizure in childhood: a prospective study. *Pediatrics,* **85,** 1076-1085.

Sillanpää M. (1993). Remission of seizures and predictors of intractability in long-term follow-up. *Epilepsia,* **34,** 930-936.

Sillanpää, M. (2000). Long-term outcome of epilepsy. *Epileptic Disord,* **2,** 79-88.

Sillanpää, M. (2005). Anti-epileptic drug interactions in handicapped and mentally retarded patients. In: Majkowski, J., Bourgeois, B.F.D., Patsalos, P. and Mattson, R. (Eds), *Anti-Epileptic Drugs. Combination Therapy and Interactions.* Cambridge University Press, Cambridge, pp. 325-340.

Sillanpää, M., Jalava, M., Kaleva, O. and Shinnar, S. (1998). Long-term prognosis of seizures with onset in childhood. *N Engl J Med,* **338,** 1715-1722.

Sillanpää, M., Haataja, L. and Shinnar, S. (2004). Perceived impact of childhood-onset epilepsy on quality of life as an adult. *Epilepsia,* **45,** 971-977.

Sillanpää, M. and Schmidt, D. (2006). Natural history of treated childhood-onset epilepsy: prospective, long-term population-based study. *Brain,* **129,** 617-624.

Sofijanov, N. G. (1982). Clinical evolution and prognosis of childhood epilepsies. *Epilepsia,* **23,** 61-69.

Seizure Freedom: Clinical, Research and Quality of Life Perspectives
Edited by Michael R. Trimble
© 2006 Clarius Press Ltd

2

Neuroprotection with Anti-Epileptic Drugs: State of the Evidence

ASLA PITKÄNEN[1,2]

[1] *A.I. Virtanen Institute for Molecular Sciences,
Department of Neurobiology, University of Kuopio,
Kuopio, Finland*

[2] *Department of Neurology, Kuopio University Hospital,
Kuopio, Finland.*

INTRODUCTION

The reorganisation of neuronal circuits after epileptogenic brain insults comprises several neurobiological alterations that are orchestrated in a parallel and serial manner, including neuronal and glial cell death, neurogenesis and gliogenesis, axonal and dendritic plasticity, axonal damage, vascular alterations, and remodelling of the extracellular matrix and cellular membranes (Pitkänen and Sutula, 2002). The prevention or alleviation of neurodegeneration at different phases of the epileptic process remains the most attractive target for therapeutic attempts to improve outcome (Pitkänen and Kubova, 2004).

Depending on the type of epileptogenic insult *e.g.* traumatic brain injury (TBI), status epilepticus (SE), stroke, infection, the mechanisms of damage can vary from direct mechanical forces to tissue (*e.g.* in TBI) to insult-induced excitotoxicity leading to necrosis or to apoptosis (*e.g.* in SE, stroke) triggered by the activation of death receptors, mitochondrial pathways, or possibly endoplasmic reticulum (Henshall and Simon, 2005; Pitkänen and McIntosh, 2006). Neurodegeneration related to an underlying epileptogenic insult can continue for months to years, providing a large window of opportunity for neuroprotective therapies. Inter-individual differences in the progression of brain atrophy might be related to age, genetic background, ongoing medication, or substance abuse.

Recent advances in modelling symptomatic epilepsies in rodents by using brain insults other than SE, however, have highlighted the importance of factors other than neuronal damage that should be considered when planning novel strategies to improve long-term outcome. In addition to neurons, glia (both oligodendrocytes and astrocytes), newly-born cells, axons, and blood vessels can be damaged by epileptogenic insults. The regional and cellular distribution of damage depend on the type of epileptogenic injury (Pitkänen and McIntosh, 2006). Importantly, protective treatments targeted to different cellular compartments of the circuitry can result in several beneficial functional consequences that can be achieved independently, including anti-epileptogenesis, disease modification (better behavioural and cognitive performance, less severe epilepsy, no drug-refractoriness), or prevention of developmental delay.

We review recent data that provide evidence that antiepileptic drugs (AEDs) have effects beyond the protection of neuronal somata against necrotic or apoptotic damage. Even though the data are fragmentary and available only for a subgroup of compounds, analysis of the information suggests that the effects of AEDs are not limited to the neuronal somata, but also include glia, axons, and blood vessels; thus, providing new insight as to why some AEDs might have more beneficial effects on recovery than others (Hernandez, 1997). The mechanisms of actions of AEDs seem to predict some of these properties (Table 1).

EFFECTS OF ACUTE TREATMENT WITH ANTI-EPILEPTIC DRUGS ON NEURONAL CELL DEATH IN *IN VIVO* MODELS OF EPILEPTOGENESIS

The neuroprotective effects of post-treatment with AEDs on acute neuronal damage in rats that have been exposed to epileptogenic brain insults are summarised in Table 2. The best neuroprotection and anti-epileptogenic effects are obtained by terminating SE at an early phase using various AEDs, which results in reduced acute (necrotic) neurodegeneration and a decreased percentage of rats that develop epilepsy (Lemos and Cavalheiro, 1995; Prasad et al., 2002; Brandt et al., 2003a; Pitkänen et al., 2005). Further, if epilepsy develops, the seizure frequency is milder (Pitkänen et al., 2005). The association of these effects with neuroprotection, however, was challenged by the observations of Brandt and colleagues that despite a substantial protection of hilar cells and hippocampal principal cells with NMDA receptor blockade, epileptogenesis is not prevented, and frequency of seizures is not decreased

Table 1. Mechanisms of action of anti-epileptic drugs which presumably contribute to their neuroprotective effects.

Site of action	AED
GABA$_A$ receptor	benzodiazepines
	clobazam
	clonazepam
	ganaloxolone
	phenobarbital
	primidone
	retigabine
GABA transaminase	vigabatrin
GABA transporter	tiagabine
AMPA/KA receptor	NS1209
	talampanel
	topiramate
NMDA receptor	felbamate
	fluorofelbamate
Voltage-gated Na$^+$ channel	BIA -093
	carbamazepine
	felbamate
	fluorofelbamate
	fos-phenytoin
	gabapentin
	lamotrigine
	oxcarbazepine
	phenytoin
	saffinamide
	topiramate
	valproate
	zonisamide
Voltage-gated K$^+$ channel	retigabine
Voltage-gated Ca^{2+} channel	gabapentin
	pregabalin
• N-type and/or P/Q type	lamotrigine
	oxcarbazepine
	topiramate
• L-type	felbamate
	gabapentin
	topiramate
• T-type	ethosuximide
	lamotrigine
	phenytoin
	zonisamide
Other	
• indirectly via CYP enzymes	stiripentol
• MAO-B inhibition	saffinamide
• SV2A	levetiracetam
	ucb 34714
Unknown	lacosamide
	NPS 1776
	RWJ 333369
	valrocemide

For references of mechanisms of action, see the recent review by Bialer *et al.* (2004).

Table 2.   Effect of anti-epileptic drugs (AEDs) on neuronal damage caused by brain injury associated with an elevated risk of epileptogenesis. Note that only the studies in which the AED was administered *during or after* the insult induced *in vivo* are included (for references, see text).

Drug	Status epilepticus	Ischemia	Traumatic brain injury
BIA2-093	n.d.	n.d.	n.d.
Carbamazepine	n.d.	±0 or ↓	n.d.
Clobazam	n.d.	n.d.	n.d.
Clonazepam	n.d.	↓	n.d.
Ethosuximide	n.d.	n.d.	n.d.
Felbamate*	↓	↓	n.d.
	n.d.	↓	n.d.
Fos-phenytoin	n.d.	n.d.	n.d.
Gabapentin	↓	n.d.	n.d.
Ganaxolone	n.d.	n.d.	n.d.
Lacosamide	↓	n.d.	±0
Lamotrigine	±0 or ↓	±0 or ↓	n.d.
	↓	↓	n.d.
Levetiracetam	±0 or ↓	n.d.	n.d.
NPS 1776	n.d.	n.d.	n.d.
NS1209	n.d	n.d	n.d.
Oxcarbazepine	n.d.	↓	n.d.
Phenobarbital	±0 or ↓	n.d.	n.d.
Phenytoin	n.d.	±0 or ↓	n.d.
Pregabalin	↓	n.d.	n.d.
	±0	n.d.	n.d.
Primidone	n.d.	n.d.	n.d.
Retigabine	↓	n.d.	n.d.
RWJ 333369	n.d.	n.d.	n.d.
Safinamide	n.d.	n.d.	n.d.
Stiripentol	n.d.	n.d.	n.d.
Talampanel	n.d.	n.d.	↓
Tiagabine	n.d.	±0 or ↓	n.d.
Topiramate	±0 or ↓	↓	n.d.
ucb 34714	n.d.	n.d.	n.d.
Valproate	±0 or ↓	n.d.	n.d.
Valrocemide	n.d.	n.d.	n.d.
Vigabatrin	±0 or ↓	↓	n.d.
Zonisamide	n.d.	±0 or ↓	n.d.

Abbreviations: AED, antiepileptic drug; n.d., no data available; SE, status epilepticus; ±0 no effect; ↓ reduction in the severity of damage; * includes data also from fluorofelbamate. Data are revised and updated from original presentation by Pitkänen and Kubova (2004).

(Ebert *et al.*, 2002; Brandt *et al.*, 2003b). Neuroprotective effects have been extensively studied in the hippocampus, and some studies reported beneficial effects of various treatments on hippocampus-dependent spatial memory performance (for review, see Pitkänen and Kubova, 2004). The beneficial cognitive effects, however, were not associated with anti-epileptogenic effects (see Pitkänen and Kubova, 2004).

Programmed cell death seems to be the predominant mechanism of cell degeneration at later post-injury time points when it occurs in parallel with neurogenesis, axonal injury, and angiogenesis, which also contribute to functional outcome (Narkilahti and Pitkänen, 2003). We review the available data on the effects of AEDs on apoptosis and axonal damage. Also, we briefly summarise recent molecular profiling studies that provide evidence that AEDs also affect reshaping of the extracellular matrix and blood vessels.

ANTI-APOPTOTIC EFFECTS OF ANTI-EPILEPTIC DRUGS

The effects of AEDs on apoptosis in *in vitro* and *in vivo* models are summarised in Table 3. The protective or apoptotic effects seem to vary depending on the mechanisms of action and the dose of each AED, as well as the cell culture preparation used or the age of the animal at the time of exposure. The best results are obtained using compounds that block sodium channels, even though some of these compounds are clearly pro-apoptotic in cell culture models.

AEDs with effects on Na+ channels

Valproic acid (0-2 mM) protects cultured cerebellar granule cells against low K+-induced apoptosis by acting on the phosphatidylinositol 3-kinase/protein kinase B pathway (Mora *et al.*, 1999). There are no effects, however, on caspase 3 activation (Mora *et al.*, 2002). Valproate also protects human neuroblastoma SH-SY5Y cells by inhibiting the pro-apoptotic effects of glycogen synthase kinase-3β (Li *et al.*, 2002). The histone deacetylase inhibition effect of valproate as well as the protection against calcium release from the endoplasmic reticulum are likely associated with its anti-apoptotic effect (Chuang, 2005). Recently, Bittigau *et al.*, (2002) reported that the administration of valproate to immature rats (50-400 mg/kg, twice a day for three days) caused apoptosis in a dose-dependent manner in various cortical and subcortical areas. Similar to the effects of phenytoin, increased apoptosis was proposed to be related to depressed synthesis of neurotrophins and reduced levels of survival proteins. Like valproate, lamotrigine protects human neuroblastoma SH-SY5Y cells by inhibiting the pro-apoptotic effects of glycogen synthase kinase-3β (Li *et al.*, 2002).

Table 3.   Effect of anti-epileptic drugs (AEDs) on apoptosis in models not associated with prolonged seizure activity.

AED	Effect	Model	Reference
BIA 2-093	↑	hippocampal neuronal cultures	Ambrosio *et al.* (2000)
carbamazepine	↑	cerebellar granule cells	Gao *et al.* (1995)
	↑	cerebellar granule cells	Nonaka *et al.* (1998)
	↑	hippocampal neuronal cultures	Ambrosio *et al.* (2000)
	±0	human neuroblastoma cells	Li *et al.* (2002)
clobazam	nd	nd	nd
clonazepam	↑	immature brain	Bittigau *et al.* (2002)
	±0	rat C6 glioma cells	Chelli *et al.* (2004)
ethosuximide	nd	nd	nd
felbamate	nd	nd	nd
fluoro-felbamate	nd	nd	nd
gabapentin	nd	nd	nd
ganaxolone	nd	nd	nd
lacosamide	nd	nd	nd
lamotrigine	↓	human neuroblastoma cells	Li *et al.* (2002)
levetiracetam	nd	nd	nd
NPS 1776	nd	nd	nd
NS1209	nd	nd	nd
oxcarbazepine	↑	hippocampal neuronal cultures	Ambrosio *et al.* (2000)
phenobarbital	↑	immature brain	Bittigau *et al.* (2002)
phenytoin	↑	cerebellar granule cells	Yan *et al.*(1995)
	↑	cerebellar granule cells	Nonaka *et al.* (1998)
	↑	cerebellar granule cells	Zhao *et al.* (2003)
	↑	immature brain	Ohmori *et al.* (1999)
	↑	immature brain	Bittigau *et al.* (2002)
	↑	immature brain	Ogura *et al.* (2002)
fos-phenytoin	nd	nd	nd
pregabalin	nd	nd	nd
primidone	nd	nd	nd
retigabine	nd	nd	nd
RWJ 333369	nd	nd	nd
safinamide	nd	nd	nd
stiripentol	nd	nd	nd
talampanel	nd	nd	nd
tiagabine	nd	nd	nd
topiramate	↑	immature brain	Glier *et al.* (2004)
ucb 34714	nd	nd	nd

Table 3. *Continued*

AED	Effect	Model	Reference
valproate	↓	cerebellar granule cells	Mora *et al.* (1999)
	↓	human neuroblastoma cells	Mora *et al.* (2002)
	↓	human neuroblastoma cells	
	↑	immature brain	Li *et al.* (2002)
			Bittigau *et al.* (2002)
valrocemide	nd	nd	nd
vigabatrin	↑	immature brain	Bittigau *et al.* (2002)
zonisamide	nd		

Abbreviations: EAE, experimental allergic encephalomyelitis. ↑, increased apoptosis; ↓, decreased apoptosis; ±0, no effect; nd, no data available.

Yan *et al.* (1995) exposed cultured cerebellar granule cells to clinically relevant concentrations of phenytoin and reported that apoptosis was dependent on the concentration of phenytoin and time of treatment. This observation was confirmed by Nonaka *et al.* (1998) using only 20 μM phenytoin. Molecular pathways involved in phenytoin-induced cerebellar granule cell apoptosis *in vitro* include activation of c-Jun and suppression of the activity of the p44/42 extracellular signal-regulated kinase (ERK) pathway (Zhao *et al.*, 2003). Oral administration of phenytoin (35 mg/kg) to newborn mice once a day on post-natal days 2-4 causes death and impairs proliferation and migration of cerebellar granule cells and compromises dendritic growth of Purkinje cells (Ohmori *et al.*, 1999). More recently, studies on the hippocampus demonstrated transferase-mediated dUTP nick-end labelling-positive cells and thinning of the granule cell layer in the dentate gyrus, suggesting that exposure of newborn mice to phenytoin interferes with the development of granule cells (Ogura *et al.*, 2002). Degeneration of neurons by apoptotic mechanisms in various subcortical and cortical regions, including hippocampus proper and dentate gyrus, was recently demonstrated in immature rats exposed to clinically relevant doses of phenytoin twice a day for three days (Bittigau *et al.*, 2002). Apoptosis *in vivo* was proposed to be related to the depressed synthesis of neurotrophins (brain-derived neurotrophic factor, neurotrophin-3) as well as to reduced levels of active phosphorylated forms of survival proteins (c-RAF, ERK 1/2, AKT).

Gao *et al.* (1995) reported that apoptosis in cultured cerebellar granule cells treated with carbamazepine could be blocked by NMDA and cycloheximide. Nonaka *et al.* (1998) recently confirmed the observations by treating cerebellar granule cells with 100 μM carbamazepine. A 24-h exposure of hippocampal primary cell cultures to carbamazepine (100 or 300 μM, but not 50 μM) enhances apoptosis and increases caspase-3 activity (Ambrosio *et al.*, 2000). Exposure of cultures to 50 to 300 μM oxcarbazepine was even more deleterious (Ambrosio *et al.*, 2000). The new carbamazepine derivative, BIA 2-093, at 50-300 μM, is less toxic (Ambrosio *et al.*, 2000). Unlike valproate and lamotrigine, carbamazepine does not protect human neuroblastoma SH-SY5Y cells from glycogen synthase kinase-3ß -induced apoptosis (Li *et al.*, 2002).

AEDs with effects on AMPA-receptors

Glier *et al.* (2004) investigated the effects of topiramate on apoptosis in immature brain. Immature rats were exposed to a single dose of topiramate (5-80 mg/kg) and killed within 48 h. There was a slight, but significant, increase in apoptosis. As compared to phenytoin, valproate, and phenobarbital, however, the difference between the anticonvulsant and apoptosis-inducing dose of topiramate was larger than that of other AEDs.

AEDs that enhance GABAergic inhibition

Few studies have investigated the effects of phenobarbital on apoptosis. Bittigau *et al.* (2002) demonstrated that the administration of phenobarbital (20-100 mg/kg, b.i.d. for 3 days) causes apoptosis in a dose-dependent manner in various cortical and subcortical areas in immature rats. Clonazepam binding to peripheral benzodiazepine receptors located between the inner and outer mitochondrial membranes did not induce apoptosis, unlike specific peripheral benzodiazepine receptor ligands in rat C6 glioma cells (Chelli *et al.*, 2004). Administration of clonazepam to immature rats (0.5-4 mg/kg) triggers apoptosis in both cortical and subcortical areas (Bittigau *et al.*, 2002). Administration of vigabatrin to immature rats (50-200 mg/kg) triggers apoptosis in both cortical and subcortical areas (Bittigau *et al.*, 2002).

EFFECTS OF ANTI-EPILEPTIC DRUGS ON AXONAL INJURY

Various epileptogenic brain insults in experimental models and in humans, including TBI, stroke, and SE, are associated with axonal injury (Meller *et al.*, 1993; Pantoni *et al.*, 1996; Reichard *et al.*, 2005). Studies designed to understand the mechanisms of axonal injury demonstrate the importance of sodium channels and AMPA-receptors as candidate targets to alleviate axonal injury (Stys, 2005). As summarised in Table 4, several AEDs affecting these receptors or channels are protective in *in vitro* and *in vivo* models of axonal injury.

AEDs with effects on Na^+ channels

Tetrodotoxin-sensitive Na^+ channels (particularly Nav1.6) are expressed in the nodes of Ranvier of myelinated axons and along unmyelinated axons (Caldwell *et al.*, 2000). During traumatic conditions, Na^+ influx through voltage-dependent Na^+ channels associated with depolarisation causes the Na^+- Ca^{2-} exchanger to operate in reverse, thereby imposing a lethal axoplasmic Ca^{2+} overload (Stys, 2005). The signalling mechanisms that eventually lead to axonal injury are poorly understood. Iwata *et al.* (2004) demonstrated that mechanical trauma of axons and Na^+ influx through tetrodotoxin-sensitive Na^+ channels triggers initial increases in intracellular Ca^{2+} and subsequent proteolysis of the Na^+ channel-α subunit. Degradation of the α-subunit promotes persistent elevations in intracellular Ca^{2+}, exposing the axons to additional pathological changes. Nav1.6 contains a putative MAP-kinase recognition module in the intracellular loop, which might be another mechanism mediating axonal injury (Wittmack *et al.*, 2005). As discussed below, Na^+ channels have a significant role in the optic nerve (anoxia, glucose-oxygen (G/O) deprivation) and spinal cord (anoxia, contusion) models of axonal injury.

The protective effects of several Na$^+$ channel blockers with anti-epileptic efficacy, including phenytoin, carbamazepine, valproic acid, and lamotrigine, have been tested against axonal injury in experimental models. The application of phenytoin and carbamazepine at concentrations lower than those used to treat seizures in optic nerve preparations exposed to 60 minutes of anoxia results in substantial recovery of the axon potential [60% and 54%, respectively compared to that of vehicle (35%)] (Fern *et al.*, 1993). Phenytoin and carbamazepine also improve recovery of the amplitude of the axon potential in a spinal cord anoxia model (Imaizumi *et al.*, 1997). In a model in which 50% of the optic nerve axons degenerate within approximately one month after neuro—inflammation (experimental allergic encephalomyelitis, EAE), administration of phenytoin alleviates the damage to only 12% (Lo *et al.*, 2002). In a mouse spinal cord model of EAE, phenytoin administration started 10 days after the induction of EAE at a dose that results in anti-epileptic plasma concentrations reduced axonal degeneration in the dorsal column (from 43% to 17%) and dorsal corticospinal tract (from 63% to 28%)(Lo *et al.*, 2003). Hains *et al.* (2004) started chronic oral treatment with an anti-epileptic dose of phenytoin three days before induction of a T9 contusion of the spinal cord in rats. Immunohistochemical analysis of the axons indicated significant axon sparing for up to eight weeks post-injury. A recent electron-microscopic study by Kaptanoglu *et al.* (2005) demonstrated that intraperitoneal injection of phenytoin (30 mg/kg) immediately after weight drop-induced spinal cord contusion protects axons and myelin when assessed hours post-injury. Lower phenytoin doses, however, had no effect.

There are also some data available on the protective effects of valproate and lamotrigine on axonal injury. Cui *et al.* (2003) reported that valproate alleviated the damage and improved the functional outcome after sciatic nerve axotomy in rat. Garthwite and colleagues (1999a) investigated the neuroprotective effects of lamotrigine in rat optic nerve axons in which degeneration was induced by glucose and oxygen deprivation. Analysis of biochemical and histological markers indicated that 100 mM lamotrigine provided a 40% to 50% protection against glucose and oxygen deprivation-induced axonal injury. Electron-microscopic analysis of the axon morphology confirmed these observations (Garthwite *et al.*, 1999b).

AEDs with effects on AMPA-receptors

AMPA-receptors are located in the myelin sheath and in oligodendrocytes that produce myelin and provide trophic support for axons (see Rosin *et al.*, 2004). Therefore, it is not surprising that AMPA receptor activation contributes to white matter damage in various experimental conditions in mature and immature brain (Rosin *et al.*, 2004). Further, administration of AMPA/kainate receptor antagonists (*e.g.*, NBQX, GYKI 52466, or EGIS

10608) reduces oligodendrocyte death and white matter damage in spinal cord ischaemia and contusion models (Kanellopoulos *et al.,* 2000; Styss, 2005), an impact acceleration model of TBI (Goda *et al.,* 2002), AMPA agonist (S-bromo-willardiine) –induced brain damage *in vivo* in newborn mice (postnatal day 5) (Gressens *et al.,* 2005), and oligodendrocyte death induced by G/O deprivation in cell cultures and in slice preparations (McDonald *et al.,* 1998; Fern and Möller, 2000; Yoshika *et al.,* 2000; Tekkök and Goldberg, 2001; Tekkök *et al.,* 2005). Even though downstream cascades mediating the damage are poorly understood, the possibility to affect white matter damage via AMPA receptors provides a target that can be modulated to alleviate neurodegeneration after epileptogenic insults by using novel compounds, including some AEDs (Table 4).

There are currently three AEDs with AMPA receptor activity, NS1209, talampanel, and topiramate (Table 1). Intravenous administration of a novel specific AMPA-receptor antagonist, NS1209, before and during transient medial cerebral artery occlusion in adult rats reduced damage to myelinated tracts by 45% when assessed 24 h post-injury. Particularly, the cortical oligo-dendrocyte damage was reduced by 53% (McCracken *et al.,* 2002).

Two studies addressed the protective effects of topiramate on white matter damage in immature brain. Follet and coworkers (2004) reported that topira-mate reduced kainate-induced pre-oligodendrocyte death *in vitro*. Further, the administration of topiramate (30 mg/kg) reduced subcortical white matter damage in P7 rats exposed to hypoxic-ischaemic injury *in vivo* (a model of periventricular leucomalasia) when assessed from myelin basic protein–stained preparations. Sfaello and colleagues (2005) investigated the protective effects of topiramate on white matter damage that was induced by intracerebral administration of S-bromo-willardiine (acting on AMPA recep-tors) to rats on postnatal day 5. Topiramate administration reduced both the white matter damage in myelin basic protein-stained sections as well as pre-oligodendrocyte damage (O4 immunostaining). As oligodendrocytes do not express tetrodotoxin-sensitive Na^+ channels, it is not surprising that sodium channel blockers (phenytoin or carbamazepine) did not alleviate oligoden-drocyte damage in the same experimental paradigm.

AEDs that enhance GABAergic inhibition

Harmful effects of vigabatrin on white matter in immature rats were demon-strated by Sidhu *et al.* (1997). They administered clinically relevant doses of vigabatrin to immature rats for four days starting at P12. In addition to axonal degeneration, there was glial cell death in white matter as well as delayed myelination. The effects of other compounds that primarily affect the GABAergic system on axonal injury or oligodendrocyte survival have not been examined.

Table 4.   Effect of anti-epileptic drugs (AEDs) on experimental axonal injury.

AED	Effect	Model	Reference
BIA 2-093	nd	nd	nd
carbamazepine	↓	rat optic nerve anoxic injury	Fern *et al.* (1993)
	↓	rat optic nerve anoxic injury	Styss *et al.* (1995)
	±0	white matter damage in newborn	Sfaello *et al.* (2005)
clobazam	nd	nd	nd
clonazepam	nd	nd	nd
ethosuximide	nd	nd	nd
felbamate*	nd	nd	nd
gabapentin	nd	nd	nd
ganaxolone	nd	nd	nd
lacosamide	nd	nd	nd
lamotrigine	↓	rat optic nerve axonl injury (GOD)	Garthwaite *et al.* (1999a, b)
levetiracetam	nd	nd	nd
NPS 1776	nd	nd	nd
NS1209	↓	MCA occlusion in rat	McCracken *et al.* (2002)
oxcarbazepine	nd	nd	nd
phenobarbital	nd	nd	nd
phenytoin	↑	purkinje cell axons	Kiefer *et al.* (1989)
	↑	cultured purkinje cell axons	Taner *et al.* (1998)
	↓	rat optic nerve anoxic injury	Fern *et al.* (1993)
	↓	spinal cord injury	Schwartz *et al.* (2001)
	↓	spinal cord injury	Hains *et al.* (2004)
	↓	spinal cord injury	Kaptanoglu *et al.* (2005)
	↓	axon loss in EAE	Lo *et al.* (2002)
	±0	white matter damage in newborn	Sfaello *et al.* (2005)
fos-phenytoin	nd	nd	nd
pregabalin	nd	nd	nd
primidone	nd	nd	nd
retigabine	nd	nd	nd
RWJ 333369	nd	nd	nd
safinamide	nd	nd	nd
stiripentol	nd	nd	nd
talampanel	nd	nd	nd
tiagabine	nd	nd	nd
topiramate	↓	white matter damage	Follett *et al.* (2004)
	↓	white matter damage	Sfaello *et al.* (2005)
ucb 34714	nd	nd	nd
valproate	↓	sciatic nerve axotomy	Cui *et al.* (2003)

Table 4.   *Continued*

AED	Effect	Model	Reference
valrocemide	nd	nd	nd
vigabatrin	↑	white matter damage in immature rats	Sidhu *et al.* (1997)
zonisamide	nd	nd	nd

Abbreviations: GOD, glucose-oxygen deprivation; EAE, experimental allergic encephalomyelitis;
MCA, medial cerebral artery. ↑, increased damage; ↓, alleviation of damage; ±0, no effect; nd, no data available.
 * includes fluoro-felbamate (no data available).

OTHER POSSIBLE EFFECTS OF ANTI-EPILEPTIC DRUGS
ON THE RECOVERY PROCESS

Large scale molecular profiling studies have provided opportunities to discover new mechanisms of actions of AEDs that extend beyond their anti-epileptic effects and can mediate their effects on neuronal recovery after epileptogenic insults. So far, such analyses have been performed with tissues exposed to valproic acid, lamotrigine, or phenytoin. Bosetti *et al.* (2005) administered 200 mg/kg of valproic acid to rats for 30 days and reported that 87 of 8799 genes on an U34A Affymetrix oligonucleotide microarray were down-regulated and 35 were up-regulated. The regulated genes affect a variety of molecular pathways, including synaptic transmission; ion channels and transport; G-protein signalling; lipid, glucose, and amino acid metabolism; transcriptional and translational regulation; phosphoinositol cycle; protein kinases and phosphatases; and apoptosis. The effects on these pathways can explain some of the effects of valproic acid on psychiatric conditions as well as on the recovery process after epileptogenic brain insults. One of the effects might be on angiogenesis and cell proliferation. Interestingly, valproic acid (0.25-1 mM) was recently reported to inhibit endothelial cell proliferation and migration as well as reduce angiogenesis *in vitro* and *in vivo*, effects that are probably mediated by the inhibition of histone deacetylase and decreased expression of endothelial nitric-oxide synthase (Michaelis *et al.*, 2004). Suppressed expression of the angiogenic factors vascular endothelial growth factor and fibroblast growth factor is also proposed to contribute to the anti-angiogenic effects of valproate (Zgouras *et al.*, 2004). The effect on cellular proliferation has sparked interest in valproate as an anti-cancerogenic agent (Blaheta *et al.*, 2005). Whether trauma or seizure-induced proliferation of neuronal and glial cells is affected by valproic acid is unknown.

Wang and colleagues (2002) exposed hippocampal primary cell cultures to 0.1 mM lamotrigine for one week. Of 1200 genes on the Atlas Rat 1.2 array, eight genes were up-regulated and six were down-regulated. Regulated genes included subunits of ion channel receptors, kinases, phosphatases, and proteins involved in cell survival. The functional significance of the data has not yet been explored.

The effects of phenytoin on gene expression were studied in human dermal fibroblasts by Swamy *et al.* (2004). Of the 18,000 elements on the cDNA microarrays, 1,500 genes were differentially expressed after exposure of cultures to 20 µg/ml phenytoin for up to 48 h. Particularly, the major growth factors and their receptors involved in wound healing were up-regulated, as were the genes encoding proteins involved in extracellular matrix degradation (*e.g.* matrix metalloproteinase-1). These findings suggest a molecular basis for some peripheral effects of phenytoin, including its beneficial effects on wound healing. They are also consistent with earlier studies demonstrating that in an experimental model of wound healing, as well as in stroke patients with peripheral ulcers, phenytoin facilitates fibroblast infiltration and neovascularisation (DaCosta *et al.,* 1998; Pitiakoudis *et al.,* 2004). Further investigation of the effects of phenytoin on genes encoding proteins that contribute to the reorganisation of the extracellular matrix and blood vessels in neuronal tissue after brain trauma is necessary.

CONCLUSIONS AND FUTURE CHALLENGES

Recent observations indicate that the prevention of cellular degeneration is a multifaceted task that requires the interference of multiple mechanisms, perhaps in a parallel and serial manner. Further, neuroprotection should be expanded to include not only the protection of somata exposed to damaging mechanisms, but also glia, newly born cells, axons, and blood vessels. In this scenario, interfering with neuronal necrosis or apoptosis might be too limited of an approach when aiming at improving the different aspects of functional outcome during the epileptic process. The experimental data suggest that many AEDs have beneficial effects on epilepsy beyond seizure suppression. Many of these effects, however, have not been systematically investigated. It is time to expand our view of neuroprotection to brain protection, and to evaluate the overall effects of AEDs on circuitry reorganisation after epileptogenic brain insult.

REFERENCES

Ambrosio, A. F., Silva, A. P., Araujo, I., Malva, J. O., Soares-da-Silva, P., Carvalho, A. P., and Carvalho, C. M. (2000). Neurotoxic/neuroprotective profile of carbamazepine, oxcarbazepine and two new putative antiepileptic drugs, BIA 2-093 and BIA 2-024. *Eur J Pharmacol* **406**, 191-201.

Bialer, M., Johannessen, S. I., Kupferberg, H. J., Levy, R. H., Perucca, E., and Tomson, T. (2004). Progress report on new antiepileptic drugs: a summary of the Seventh Eilat Conference (EILAT VII). *Epilepsy Res* **61**, 1-48.

Bittigau, P., Sifringer, M., Genz, K., Reith, E., Pospischil, D., Govindarajalu, S., Dzietko, M., Pesditschek, S., Mai, I., Dikranian, K., *et al.* (2002). Antiepileptic drugs and apoptotic neurodegeneration in the developing brain. *Proc Natl Acad Sci USA* **99**, 15089-15094.

Blaheta, R. A., Michaelis, M., Driever, P. H., and Cinatl, J., Jr. (2005). Evolving anticancer drug valproic acid: insights into the mechanism and clinical studies. *Med Res Rev* **25**, 383-397.

Bosetti, F., Bell, J. M., and Manickam, P. (2005). Microarray analysis of rat brain gene expression after chronic administration of sodium valproate. *Brain Res Bull* **65**, 331-338.

Brandt, C., Glien, M., Potschka, H., Volk, H., and Löscher, W.A. (2003a). Epileptogenesis and neuropathology after different types of status epilepticus induced by prolonged electrical stimulation of the basolateral amygdala in rats. *Epilepsy Res* **55**, 83-103.

Brandt, C., Potschka, H., Loscher, W., and Ebert, U. (2003b). N-methyl-D-aspartate receptor blockade after status epilepticus protects against limbic brain damage but not against epilepsy in the kainate model of temporal lobe epilepsy. *Neuroscience* **118(3)**, 727-740.

Caldwell, J.H., Schaller, K.L., Lasher, R.S., Peles, E., and Levinson, S.R. (2000) Sodium channel Na(v)1.6 is localized at nodes of ranvier, dendrites, and synapses. *Proc Natl Acad Sci USA* **97(10)**, 5616-5620.

Chelli, B., Lena, A., Vanacore, R., Pozzo, E. D., Costa, B., Rossi, L., Salvetti, A., Scatena, F., Ceruti, S., Abbracchio, M. P., *et al.* (2004). Peripheral benzodiazepine receptor ligands: mitochondrial transmembrane potential depolarization and apoptosis induction in rat C6 glioma cells. *Biochem Pharmacol* **68**, 125-134.

Chuang, D. M. (2005). The Antiapoptotic Actions of Mood Stabilizers: Molecular Mechanisms and Therapeutic Potentials. *Ann N Y Acad Sci* **1053**, 195-204.

Cui, S. S., Yang, C. P., Bowen, R. C., Bai, O., Li, X. M., Jiang, W., and Zhang, X. (2003). Valproic acid enhances axonal regeneration and recovery of motor function after sciatic nerve axotomy in adult rats. *Brain Res* **975**, 229-236.

DaCosta, M. L., Regan, M. C., al Sader, M., Leader, M., and Bouchier-Hayes, D. (1998). Diphenylhydantoin sodium promotes early and marked angiogenesis and results in increased collagen deposition and tensile strength in healing wounds. *Surgery* **123**, 287-293.

Ebert, U., Brandt, C., and Löscher, W. (2002). Delayed sclerosis, neuroprotection, and limbic epileptogenesis after status epilepticus in the rat. *Epilepsia* **43(Suppl 5)**, S86-S95.

Fern, R., Ransom, B. R., Stys, P. K., and Waxman, S. G. (1993). Pharmacological protection of CNS white matter during anoxia: actions of phenytoin, carbamazepine and diazepam. *J Pharmacol Exp Ther* **266**, 1549-1555.

Fern, R. and Möller, T. (2000). Rapid ischemic cell death in immature oligodendrocytes: a fatal glutamate release feedback loop. *J Neurosci* **20**, 34-42.

Follett, P. L., Deng, W., Dai, W., Talos, D. M., Massillon, L. J., Rosenberg, P. A., Volpe, J. J., and Jensen, F. E. (2004). Glutamate receptor-mediated oligodendrocyte toxicity in periventricular leukomalacia: a protective role for topiramate. *J Neurosci* **24**, 4412-4420.

Gao, X. M., Margolis, R. L., Leeds, P., Hough, C., Post, R. M., and Chuang, D. M. (1995). Carbamazepine induction of apoptosis in cultured cerebellar neurons: effects of N-methyl-D-aspartate, aurintricarboxylic acid and cycloheximide. *Brain Res* **703**, 63-71.

Garthwaite, G., Goodwin, D. A., and Garthwaite, J. (1999a). Nitric oxide stimulates cGMP formation in rat optic nerve axons, providing a specific marker of axon viability. *Eur J Neurosci* **11**, 4367-4372.

Garthwaite, G., Brown, G., Batchelor, A. M., Goodwin, D. A., and Garthwaite, J. (1999b). Mechanisms of ischaemic damage to central white matter axons: a quantitative histological analysis using rat optic nerve. *Neuroscience* **94**, 1219-1230.

Glier, C., Dzietko, M., Bittigau, P., Jarosz, B., Koroboicz, E., and Ikonomidou, C. (2004). Therapeutic doses of topiramate are not toxic to the developing rat brain. *Exp Neurol* **187**, 403-409.

Goda, M., Isono, M., Fujiki, M., and Kobayashi, H. (2002). Both MK801 and NBQX reduce the neuronal damage after impact-acceleration brain injury. *J Neurotrauma* **19**, 1445-1456.

Gressens, P., Spedding, M., Gigler, G., Kertesz, S., Villa, P., Medja, F., Williamson, T., Kapus, G., Levay, G., Szenasi, G., *et al.* (2005). The effects of AMPA receptor antagonists in models of stroke and neurodegeneration. *Eur J Pharmacol* **519**, 58-67.

Hains, B. C., Saab, C. Y., Lo, A. C., and Waxman, S. G. (2004). Sodium channel blockade with phenytoin protects spinal cord axons, enhances axonal conduction, and improves functional motor recovery after contusion SCI. *Exp Neurol* **188**, 365-377.

Henshall, D.C., Simon, R.P. (2005) Epilepsy and apoptosis pathways. *J Cereb Blood Flow Metab* **25(12)**, 1557-1572.

Hernandez, T.D. (1997) Preventing post-traumatic epilepsy after brain injury: weighting costs and benefits of anticonvulsant prophylaxis. *Trends Pharmacol Sci* **18**, 59-62.

Imaizumi, T., Kocsis, J. D., and Waxman, S. G. (1997). Anoxic injury in the rat spinal cord: pharmacological evidence for multiple steps in Ca(2+)-dependent injury of the dorsal columns. *J Neurotrauma* **14**, 299-311.

Iwata, A., Stys, P.K., Wolf, J.A., Chen, X.H., Taylor, A.G., Meaney, D.F., and Smith, D.H. (2004). Traumatic axonal injury induces proteolytic cleavage of the voltage-gated sodium channels modulated by tetrodotoxin and protease inhibitors. *J Neurosci* **24(19)**, 4605-4613.

Kanellopoulos, G. K., Xu, X. M., Hsu, C. Y., Lu, X., Sundt, T. M., and Kouchoukos, N. T. (2000). White matter injury in spinal cord ischemia: protection by AMPA/kainate glutamate receptor antagonism. *Stroke* **31**, 1945-1952.

Kaptanoglu, E., Solaroglu, I., Surucu, H. S., Akbiyik, F., and Beskonakli, E. (2005). Blockade of sodium channels by phenytoin protects ultrastructure and attenuates lipid peroxidation in experimental spinal cord injury. *Acta Neurochir (Wien)* **147**, 405-412 (discussion 412).

Kiefer, R., Knoth, R., Anagnostopoulos, J., and Volk, B. (1989). Cerebellar injury due to phenytoin. Identification and evolution of Purkinje cell axonal swellings in deep cerebellar nuclei of mice. *Acta Neuropathol (Berl)* **77**, 289-298.

Lemos, T. and Cavalheiro, E.A. (1995). Suppression of pilocarpine-induced status epilepticus and the late development of epilepsy in rats. *Exp Brain Res* **102**, 423-428.

Li, X., Bijur, G. N., and Jope, R. S. (2002). Glycogen synthase kinase-3beta, mood stabilizers, and neuroprotection. *Bipolar Disord* **4**, 137-144.

Lo, A. C., Black, J. A., and Waxman, S. G. (2002). Neuroprotection of axons with phenytoin in experimental allergic encephalomyelitis. *Neuroreport* **13**, 1909-1912.

Lo, A. C., Saab, C. Y., Black, J. A., and Waxman, S. G. (2003). Phenytoin protects spinal cord axons and preserves axonal conduction and neurological function in a model of neuroinflammation *in vivo*. *J Neurophysiol* **90**, 3566-3571.

McCracken, E., Fowler, J. H., Dewar, D., Morrison, S., and McCulloch, J. (2002). Grey matter and white matter ischemic damage is reduced by the competitive AMPA receptor antagonist, SPD 502. *J Cereb Blood Flow Metab* **22**, 1090-1097.

McDonald, J.W., Althomsons, S.P., Hyrc, K.L., Choi, D.W., and Goldberg, M.P. (1998). Oligodendrocytes from forebrain are highly vulnerable to AMPA/kainate-receptor -mediated excitotoxicity. *Nat Med* **4**, 291-297.

Meller, D., Bellander, B. M., Schmidt-Kastner, R., and Ingvar, M. (1993). Immunohistochemical studies with antibodies to neurofilament proteins on axonal damage in experimental focal lesions in rat. *J Neurol Sci* **117**, 164-174.

Michaelis, M., Michaelis, U. R., Fleming, I., Suhan, T., Cinatl, J., Blaheta, R. A., Hoffmann, K., Kotchetkov, R., Busse, R., Nau, H., and Cinatl, J., Jr. (2004). Valproic acid inhibits angiogenesis *in vitro* and *in vivo*. *Mol Pharmacol* **65**, 520-527.

Mora, A., Gonzalez-Polo, R. A., Fuentes, J. M., Soler, G., and Centeno, F. (1999). Different mechanisms of protection against apoptosis by valproate and Li+. *Eur J Biochem* **266**, 886-891.

Mora, A., Sabio, G., Alonso, J. C., Soler, G., and Centeno, F. (2002). Different dependence of lithium and valproate on PI3K/PKB pathway. *Bipolar Disord* **4**, 195-200.

Narkilahti, S., Pirttilä, T., Lukasiuk, K., Tuunanen, J., and Pitkänen, A. (2003) Expression and activation of caspase 3 following status epilepticus in the rat. *Eur J Neurosci* **18(6)**, 1486-1496.

Nonaka, S., Katsube, N., and Chuang, D. M. (1998). Lithium protects rat cerebellar granule cells against apoptosis induced by anticonvulsants, phenytoin and carbamazepine. *J Pharmacol Exp Ther* **286**, 539-547.

Ogura, H., Yasuda, M., Nakamura, S., Yamashita, H., Mikoshiba, K., and Ohmori, H. (2002). Neurotoxic damage of granule cells in the dentate gyrus and the cerebellum and cognitive deficit following neonatal administration of phenytoin in mice. *J Neuropathol Exp Neurol* **61**, 956-967.

Ohmori, H., Ogura, H., Yasuda, M., Nakamura, S., Hatta, T., Kawano, K., Michikawa, T., Yamashita, K., and Mikoshiba, K. (1999). Developmental neurotoxicity of phenytoin on granule cells and Purkinje cells in mouse cerebellum. *J Neurochem* **72**, 1497-1506.

Pantoni, L., Garcia, J.H., and Gutierrez, J.A. (1996) Cerebral white matter is highly vulnerable to ischemia. *Stroke* **27(9)**, 1641-1646

Pitiakoudis, M., Giatromanolaki, A., Iliopoulos, I., Tsaroucha, A. K., Simopoulos, C., and Piperidou, C. (2004). Phenytoin-induced lymphocytic chemotaxis, angiogenesis and accelerated healing of decubitus ulcer in a patient with stroke. *J Int Med Res* **32**, 201-205.

Pitkänen, A. and Sutula, T. (2002). Is epilepsy a progressive disease? Prospects for new therapeutic approaches in temporal lobe epilepsy. *Lancet (Neurology)* **1**, 173-181.

Pitkänen, A. and Kubova, H. (2004). Antiepileptic drugs in neuroprotection. *Expert Opin Pharmacother* **5**, 777-798.

Pitkänen, A., Kharatishvili, I., Narkilahti, S., Lukasiuk, K., and Nissinen, J. (2005) Treatment of status epilepticus with diazepam is antiepileptogenic and disease-modifying in rat. *Epilepsy Res* **53**, 27-42.

Pitkänen, A. and McIntosh, T.K. (2006) Animal models of post-traumatic epilepsy. *J Neurotrauma* In Press.

Pitkänen, A., Longhi, L., Marklund, N., Morales, D., and McIntosh, T.K. (2006) Mechanisms of neuronal death and neuroprotective strategies after traumatic brain injury. *Drug Discovery Today* In Press.

Prasad, A., Williamson, J.M., and Bertram, E.H. (2002). Phenobarbital and MK-801, but not phenytoin, improve long-term outcome of status epilepticus. *Ann Neurol* **51**, 175-181.

Reichard, R. R., Smith, C., and Graham, D. I. (2005). The significance of beta-APP immunoreactivity in forensic practice. *Neuropathol Appl Neurobiol* **31**, 304-313.

Rosin, C., Bates, T. E., and Skaper, S. D. (2004). Excitatory amino acid induced oligodendrocyte cell death *in vitro*: receptor-dependent and -independent mechanisms. *J Neurochem* **90**, 1173-1185.

Schwartz, G., and Fehlings, M. G. (2001). Evaluation of the neuroprotective effects of sodium channel blockers after spinal cord injury: improved behavioral and neuroanatomical recovery with riluzole. *J Neurosurg* **94**, 245-256.

Sfaello, I., Baud, O., Arzimanoglou, A., and Gressens, P. (2005). Topiramate prevents excitotoxic damage in the newborn rodent brain. *Neurobiol Dis* **20**, 837-848.

Sidhu, R. S., Del Bigio, M. R., Tuor, U. I., and Seshia, S. S. (1997). Low-dose vigabatrin (gamma-vinyl GABA)-induced damage in the immature rat brain. *Exp Neurol* **144**, 400-405.

Stys, P.K. (2005). General mechanisms of axonal damage and its prevention. *J Neurol Sci* **233(1-2)**, 3-13.

Swamy, S. M., Tan, P., Zhu, Y. Z., Lu, J., Achuth, H. N., and Moochhala, S. (2004). Role of phenytoin in wound healing: microarray analysis of early transcriptional responses in human dermal fibroblasts. *Biochem Biophys Res Commun* **314**, 661-666.

Tauer, U., Knoth, R., and Volk, B. (1998). Phenytoin alters Purkinje cell axon morphology and targeting *in vitro*. *Acta Neuropathol (Berl)* **95**, 583-591.

Tekkök, S. B., and Goldberg, M. P. (2001). AMPA/kainate receptor activation mediates hypoxic oligodendrocyte death and axonal injury in cerebral white matter. *J Neurosci* **21**, 4237-4248.

Tekkök, S. B., Faddis, B. T., and Goldberg, M. P. (2005). AMPA/kainate receptors mediate axonal morphological disruption in hypoxic white matter. *Neurosci Lett* **382**, 275-279.

Wang, J. F., Sun, X., Chen, B., and Young, L. T. (2002). Lamotrigine increases gene expression of GABA-A receptor beta3 subunit in primary cultured rat hippocampus cells. *Neuropsychopharmacology* **26**, 415-421.

Wittmack, E. K., Rush, A. M., Hudmon, A., Waxman, S. G., and Dib-Hajj, S. D. (2005). Voltage-gated sodium channel Nav1.6 is modulated by p38 mitogen-activated protein kinase. *J Neurosci* **25**, 6621-6630.

Yan, G. M., Irwin, R. P., Lin, S. Z., Weller, M., Wood, K. A., and Paul, S. M. (1995). Diphenylhydantoin induces apoptotic cell death of cultured rat cerebellar granule neurons. *J Pharmacol Exp Ther* **274**, 983-990.

Yoshioka, A., Yamaya, Y., Saiki, S., Kanemoto, M.m Hirose, G., Beesley, J., and Pleasure, D. (2000). Non-N-methyl-D-aspartate glutmate receptors mediate oxygen-glucose deprivation-induced oligodendroglial injury. *Brain Res* **854**, 207-217.

Zgouras, D., Becker, U., Loitsch, S., and Stein, J. (2004). Modulation of angiogenesis-related protein synthesis by valproic acid. *Biochem Biophys Res Commun* **316**, 693-697.

Zhao, L. Z., Su, X. W., Huang, Y. J., Qiu, P. X., and Yan, G. M. (2003). Activation of c-Jun and suppression of phospho-p44/42 were involved in diphenylhydantoin-induced apoptosis of cultured rat cerebellar granule neurons. *Acta Pharmacol Sin* **24**, 539-548.

Seizure Freedom: Clinical, Research and Quality of Life Perspectives
Edited by Michael R. Trimble
© 2006 Clarius Press Ltd

3

Turning Seizures On and Off: Neurobiological Perspectives

JEROME ENGEL Jr

Departments of Neurology and Neurobiology
& the Brain Research Institute
David Geffen School of Medicine at UCLA
Los Angeles, CA, USA.

INTRODUCTION

An epileptic seizure can occur without epilepsy as a natural response of a normal brain to transient insult. These are referred to as 'acute symptomatic', 'provoked', or 'reactive' seizures. A diagnosis of epilepsy, however, implies that seizures result from an enduring epileptogenic abnormality of the brain, an inherent cerebral disturbance existing between seizures capable of initiating recurrent spontaneous ictal events (Fisher *et al.*, 2005).

Causes of epilepsy and reactive seizures are multifactorial. Three important factors are illustrated in Figure 1 (Engel, 1989). One factor determines the propensity, or threshold, in individual patients, for which ictal events are likely to be initiated. Inter-individual variation in threshold is largely genetically determined, but physical or chemical disturbances of brain structure and function also influence threshold. Threshold is not a static phenomenon, but varies in any given individual over time. For instance, there are diurnal variations in threshold related to the sleep-wake cycle, as well as monthly variations in women related to the estrous cycle. Anti-epileptic drugs exert their effect by increasing the seizure threshold.

A second factor is a specific epileptogenic abnormality, which could be a congenital or acquired structural lesion or a metabolic disturbance causing a symptomatic epilepsy, or a genetic defect giving rise to an idiopathic epilepsy. The degree of epileptogenicity of such a disturbance can also vary over time.

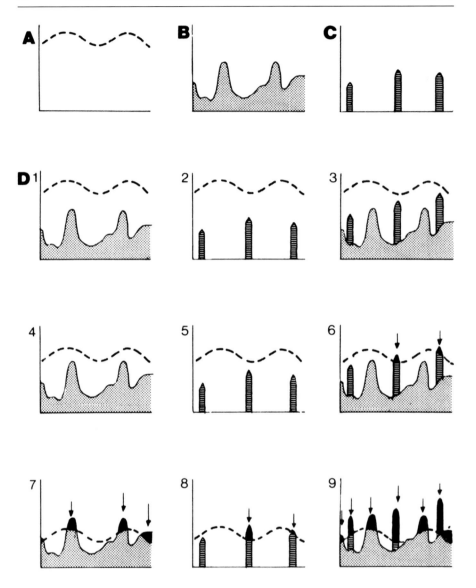

Figure 1. Schematic diagram illustrating interactions of the fluctuating threshold for seizures determined by nonspecific predisposing factors (A); independent fluctuations of a specific epileptogenic disturbance (B); and intermittent precipitating factors (C). With a high threshold, epileptogenic disturbances and precipitating factors alone (D1, D2) and combined (D3) fail to generate seizures. With an intermediate threshold, epileptogenic disturbances and precipitating factors alone (D4, D5) fail to generate seizures, but seizures (arrows) occur when these factors are combined (D6). With a low threshold, epileptogenic disturbances and precipitating factors alone (D7, D8) are each capable of generating seizures, and combined (D9) generate even more seizures, perhaps constituting status epilepticus. From Engel, 1989, with permission.

The underlying epileptogenic abnormality may require specific treatment, depending upon its nature, and if localised, it may be surgically resectable.

Finally, there are precipitating factors that can determine when an epileptic seizure occurs. In some circumstances, the precipitating factors are obvious; for instance, in reflex epilepsies, where seizures can be caused by specific sensory stimuli such as flashing lights, or acute reactive seizures provoked by head trauma, anoxic insult, or alcohol withdrawal. When precipitating factors can be identified, treatment consists of their avoidance, if possible. In most cases, however, the precipitating factors are not apparent or, perhaps, do not even exist.

As illustrated in Figure 1, if an individual is fortunate enough to have a high seizure threshold, specific epileptogenic abnormalities and precipitating factors alone, and together, may be insufficient to evoke an ictal event. If an individual is unlucky enough to have a very low seizure threshold, minor epileptogenic abnormalities can give rise to an epileptic condition, and precipitating factors alone can produce reactive seizures.

When an epileptogenic abnormality or precipitating factor is sufficient to cause seizures, regardless of the threshold, there is no single mechanism of seizure initiation. Rather, the seizure-generating pathophysiological disturbances depend upon the type of epileptogenic abnormality and precipitating factors, the anatomical area involved, and the physiological state of the brain (e.g. sleep or wake), and the resultant ictal events manifest as a variety of seizure types (Table 1) (Commission 1981; Engel, 2001). Although reactive seizures are usually generalised tonic-clonic seizures, they can also occasionally manifest as other generalised seizures such as absences or myoclonic jerks, and reactive focal seizures can occur when the threshold is lowered in a localised area of the brain due to a predisposing focal abnormality that, in itself, is not sufficient to provoke spontaneous seizures.

TURNING SEIZURES ON

The electrographic inter-ictal hallmark of most epileptic disorders is the occurrence of EEG spike and slow-wave discharges that can be bilaterally synchronous and widespread in generalised epilepsies, and localised in focal epilepsies. Experiments in animals with focal seizures induced by localised application of penicillin, which interferes with the action of the inhibitory neurotransmitter gamma amino butyric acid (GABA), show that the single-neuron correlate of the interictal EEG spike-and-wave consists of a burst of action potentials, followed by cessation of firing (Matsumoto and Ajmone-Marsan, 1964a). The membrane events underlying this abnormal neuronal bursting consists of a paroxysmal depolarisation shift (PDS) during the EEG spike, and an after-hyperpolarisation (AH) during the slow wave (Figure 2).

Table 1. Epileptic Seizure Types and Precipitating Stimuli for Reflex Seizures

Self-limited seizure types

Generalized seizures

Tonic-clonic seizures (includes variations beginning with a clonic or myoclonic phase)
Clonic seizures
        Without tonic features
        With tonic features
Typical absence seizures
Atypical absence seizures
Myoclonic absence seizures
Tonic seizures
Spasms
Myoclonic seizures
Eyelid myoclonia
        Without absences
        With absences
Myoclonic atonic seizures
Negative myoclonus
Atonic seizures

Focal seizures

Focal sensory seizures
        With elementary sensory symptoms (e.g., occipital and parietal lobe seizures)
        With experiential sensory symptoms (e.g., temporo parieto occipital junction seizures)
Focal motor seizures
        With elementary clonic motor signs
        With asymmctrical tonic motor seizures (e.g., supplementary motor seizures)
        With typical (temporal lobe) automatisms (e.g., mesial temporal lobe seizures)
        With hyperkinetic automatisms
        With focal negative myoclonus
        With inhibitory motor seizures
Gelastic seizures
Hemiclonic seizures
Secondarily generalized seizures

Continuous seizure types

Generalised status epilepticus

Generalized tonic-clonic status epilepticus
Clonic status epilepticus
Absence status epilepticus
Tonic status epilepticus
Myoclonic status epilepticus

Focal status epilepticus

Epilepsia partialis continua of Kojevnikov
Aura continua
Limbic status epilepticus (psychomotor status)
Hemiconvulsive status

Table 1.   *(continued)* Epileptic Seizure Types and Precipitating Stimuli for Reflex Seizures

Precipitating stimuli for reflex seizures

Visual stimuli
      Flickering light – color to be specified when possible
      Patterns
      Other visual stimuli
Thinking
Music
Eating
Praxis
Somatosensory
Proprioceptive
Reading
Hot water
Startle

The PDS is believed to result from abnormal calcium influx in the soma and proximal dendrites, which causes rapid sodium action potential generation at the axon hillock for as long as the PDS persists (Engel *et al.*, 1997). The PDS is reversed by the AH, which is caused by calcium-dependent potassium currents, as well as active GABA-mediated inhibition from recurrent interneuron circuits. In the penicillin focus, the PDS can be recorded in almost all neurons during the EEG spike, indicating a high degree of synchrony. Similar unit correlates can be seen with interictal spike-and-wave discharges in human epilepsy (Figure 3) (Babb and Crandall, 1976), but only a small percentage of neurons participate in these events. In contrast to the acute experimental penicillin focus, the persistent epileptogenic disturbance responsible for chronic epileptic conditions does not appear to require a large number of epileptogenically abnormal neurons.

Ictal onset in the experimental penicillin focus is characterised by a gradual disappearance of the AH and reversal to a prolonged depolarisation, causing continuous action potential generation at the axon hillock (Matsumoto and Ajmone-Marsan, 1964b). As the depolarisation gradually dissipates in one neuron, more and more adjacent neurons are recruited into this process, and the EEG shows a characteristic build-up of low-voltage fast activity (LVF), referred to as a 'recruiting rhythm' (Figure 4) (Engel *et al.*, 1997). This LVF ictal onset can be referred to as disinhibitory and appears to be the mechanism underlying the generation of generalised tonic-clonic, and some focal, seizures in patients. Generalised tonic-clonic seizures characteristically begin with a generalised recruiting rhythm on EEG (Figure 5), and many neocortical focal seizures begin with localised LVF activity. Although electrophysiological investigations have revealed the neuronal disturbances accompanying the initiation of LVF seizure types, they do not explain why loss of inhibition occurs. Precipitating factors might alter the ionic milieu, for

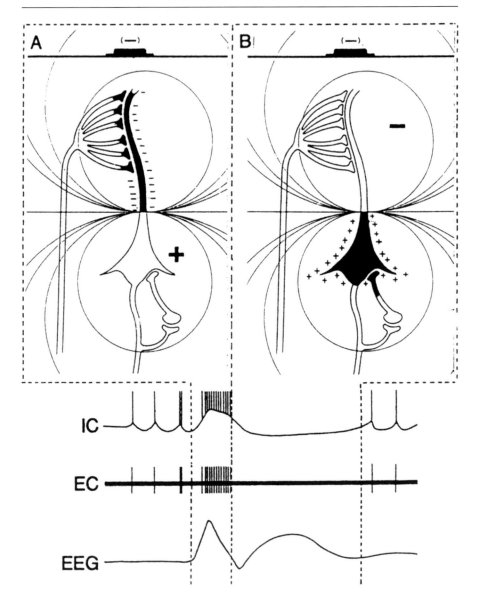

Figure 2.   Neuronal basis of the EEG spike-and-wave. A. Excitatory input opens channels on dendrite for Ca2+ entry, seen as a large PDS on intracellular recording (IC) and as burst unit firing on extracellular recording (EC). Summated outside-negative membrane events appear in the EEG as a negative spike. B. Prolonged after-hyperpolarizations caused not only by K+ currents but also by recurrent inhibition induced Cl- current at the soma are outside-positive membrane events (IC), but summate to appear as a slow negative wave in the EEG because of a dipole effect (the soma and apical dendrites maintain opposite polarity). From Engel, 1989, with permission.

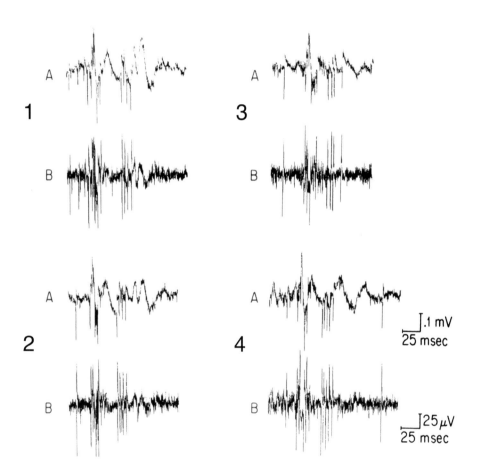

Figure 3. EEG spikes (A) and action potentials (B) recorded from the same microelectrode (63H) in the left mid-hippocampal pes (LMP) in a patient with clinical seizures originating in the LMP. Tracings 1 to 4 were taken from the beginning to the end of the recording period and selected to have a similar EEG spike morphology, characterized by a fast rise time of the initial negative component. Tracing A is a wide-band recording to show the EEG spike-and-slow-wave superimposed on the unit discharges. For tracing B, additional high-pass filtering was used to enhance the neuronal discharges. Note increased unit firing during EEG spike, and cessation of unit firing during EEG slow wave. From Babb and Crandall, 1976, with permission.

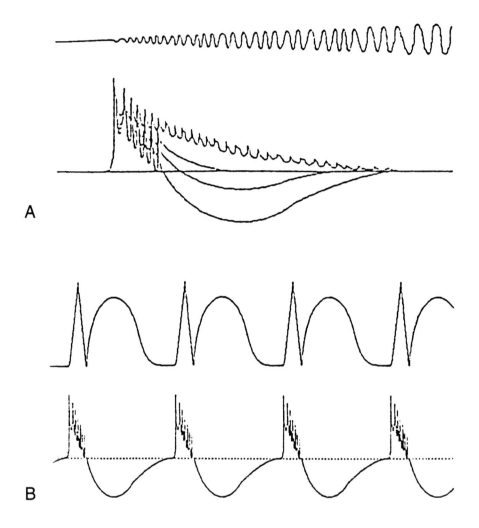

Figure 4. A. The neuronal mechanism of the recruiting rhythm shown in Figure 2A is illustrated schematically here. The lower trace represents an intracellular recording of a paroxysmal depolarisation shift (PDS), demonstrating how the afterhyperpolarization gradually disappears to become an after-depolarisation, giving rise to continuous high frequency action potential discharge. The EEG in the upper trace increases in amplitude and slows in frequency as more and more neurons are recruited into this process and develop increasing synchrony. B. The neuronal mechanism of a hypersynchronous ictal discharge, as shown in Figure 3, is schematically illustrated here. The lower trace shows an intracellular recording of recurrent PDSs. As with the interictal spike-and-wave discharge, the EEG spike, seen in the upper tracing, represents a summation of depolarization shifts, while the EEG slow wave represents a summation of after-hyperpolarisza-tions. In the ictal state, however, each hyperpolarisation is followed immediately by another PDS, creating a repetitive hypersynchronous discharge such as the classical three-per-second spike-and-wave pattern of petit mal absences. A similar mechanism appears to underlie some partial ictal events as well. From Wasterlain and Treiman, In Press, with permission.

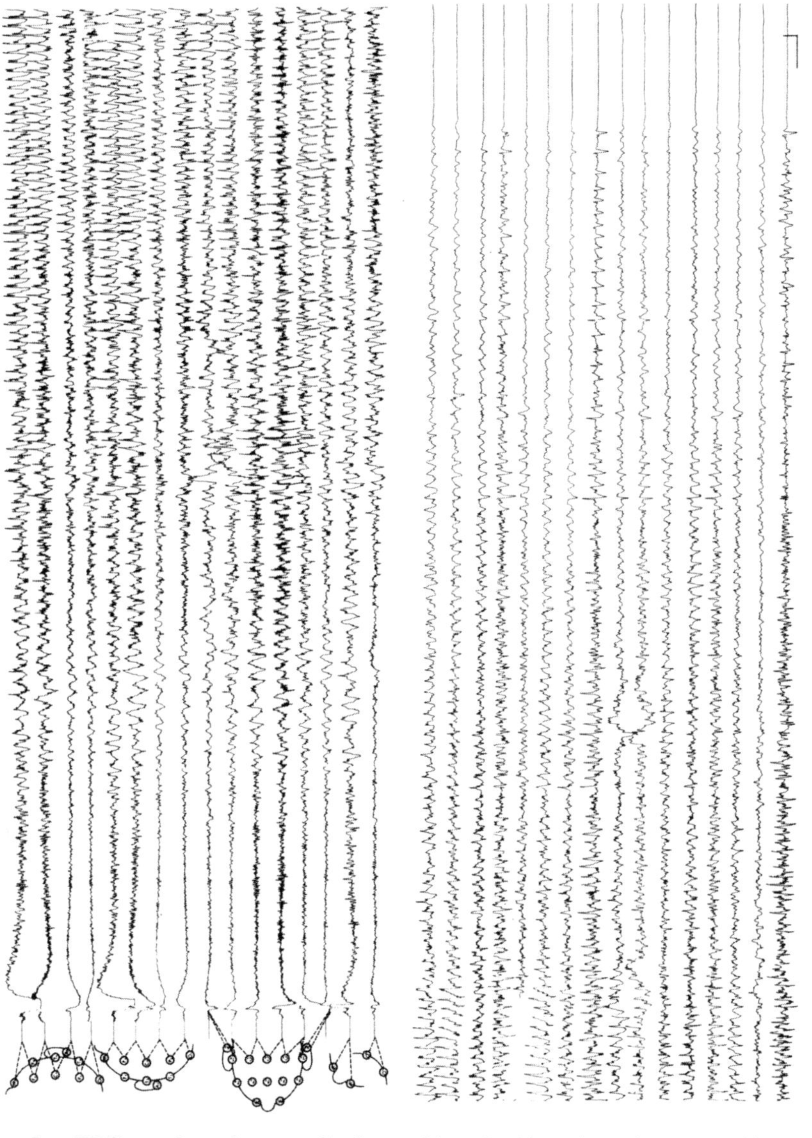

Figure 5. EEG correlate of a generalised convulsion. In this patient, electroconvulsive shock treatment (ECT) was administered under light methohexital anesthesia and mild succinylcholine paralysis. Consequently, muscle artifact is negligible. The EEG tracing begins immediately after the application of electroshock (upper left) and demonstrates a generalised recruiting rhythm, which gradually evolves into a bilaterally synchronous, 4-c/sec polyspike-and-wave pattern. The generalised polyspikes and waves first increase and then decrease in amplitude, while decreasing in frequency, and ultimately stop suddenly (bottom right), to be replaced by postictal EEG depression. The clonic phase is not particularly marked in this example, in part due to the absence of muscle artifact. Three seconds are missing between the top and bottom panels. Calibration: 1 second, 100 ?V. From Engel, 1989, with permission.

instance increasing extracellular potassium, or impair the efficacy of inhibitory synaptic influences by a variety of different mechanisms that remain poorly understood.

Seizures that begin with LVF activity usually are not static events, but evolve over time as ictal discharges propagate throughout the brain. The transition from the tonic to the clonic phase of a generalised tonic-clonic seizure, for instance, reflects propagation from brainstem and other deeper structures to the forebrain, while the transition of simple partial seizures (e.g. auras) to complex partial seizures, to secondarily generalised seizures, reflect local and long tract propagation to anatomical structures which determine the dynamic behavioural characteristics of the clinical seizure (Engel et al.,1997). It is very likely that the neuronal mechanisms underlying seizure activity at different times during this evolution vary considerably, depending on the epileptogenic abnormality and the anatomical structures involved. For some ictal events, such as generalised tonic-clonic seizures, the pathways of propagation are predetermined by normal cerebral connectivity, whereas for the focal seizures, individual differences can reflect unique pathophysiological characteristics of the specific epileptogenic abnormality, as well as normal variations in cerebral structure and function.

The concept that epileptic seizures reflect a decrease in inhibition and/or an increase in excitation by no means applies to all seizure types. The EEG correlate of typical absence seizures, for instance, consists of three-per-second spike-and-wave discharges in which the spike-and-wave of each train is identical to the interictal spike-wave discharges (Figure 6) (Engel   et al., 1997). In this case, if the slow-wave reflects the AH, this inhibitory mechanisms is not lost but, in fact, constitutes most of the ictal discharge. Electrophysiological studies in animals with experimental absence epilepsy show that the neuronal correlate of the spike of the three-per-second spike-and-wave ictal event is a PDS, and that the slow-wave is a GABA-mediated AH (Figure 4) (Giaretta et al., 1987). In this type of seizure, therefore, there is no obvious loss of inhibition, but, rather, an increase in synchronisation, which requires not only enhanced excitation, but also enhanced inhibition. Inhibition, in fact, is the mechanism the normal brain uses to synchronise neuronal populations. Absence seizures utilise the normal synchronising mechanisms of the thalamus, mediated by inhibitory input from the nucleus reticularis (McCormick and Contreras, 2001). This hyperpolarising influence de-inactivates low threshold T-type calcium currents in thalamo-cortical neurons, turning them into pacemaker cells which, under pathological conditions, synchronise the three-per-second spike-and-wave cortical discharges of absence seizures. GABAB receptor activation is believed to be responsible for the three-per-second frequency (Figure 7). Although epileptogenic abnormalities of both the cortex and the thalamus underlie absence epilepsies, ictal events appear to be initiated from the cortex.

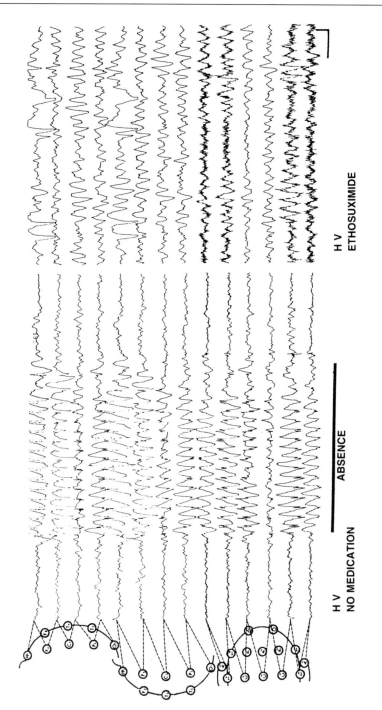

Figure 6. Left. The electroencephalographic correlate of a typical absence observed during hyperventilation prior to treatment. Right. An example of slowing that occurred during hyperventilation in the same patient several months after successful treatment with ethosuximide. Calibration: 1 second, 100 ?V. From Engel *et al.*, 1985, with permission.

Hypersynchrony (HYP) as a mechanism of seizure generation is not unique to absence seizures. Depth electrode recordings from mesial temporal structures in patients with mesial temporal lobe epilepsy demonstrate that HYP ictal onsets are much more common than LVF ictal onsets (Figure 8), and that some electrographic patterns can look very much like focal absence seizures (Figure 9) (Engel, 1988). Unlike LVF seizures, there is no evolution of typical absences, and many focal HYP ictal discharges end without evolution. Focal HYP ictal events, however, can transform into an LVF pattern, and this appears to be necessary before contralateral propagation occurs to give rise to a complex partial seizure (Engel et al.,1997). As with LVF ictal onsets, while the neuronal events associated with HYP ictal initiation are known, the precipitating factors that cause this sudden hypersynchronous onset are varied and poorly understood. These may be normal synchronising influences, for instance events that occur in association with the sleep-wake cycle, or sensory input, that are only epileptogenic when the brain is abnormally predisposed to HYP ictal discharges. Events that precipitate brief interictal spike-and-wave discharges in these conditions may be the same events that precipitate seizures, the difference being that the ictal discharges are not quickly terminated.

Recently, a unique electrophysiological feature of epileptogenic tissue called fast ripples (FR) has been identified in patients with mesial temporal lobe epilepsy, and animal models of this disorder (Figure 10) (Bragin et al.,1999a). FR are high frequency (250-600 Hz) oscillations superimposed on interictal EEG spikes, which can be recorded only from areas capable of generating spontaneous seizures. Interictal spikes outside the primary epileptogenic zone, for instance from the contralateral homotopic structures, do not demonstrate FR. Evidence suggests that FR represent the field potentials of synchronously bursting neurons, which constitute the epileptogenic substrate (Figure 11) (Bragin et al.,1999a). These bursting neurons appear to be responsible for seizure generation, because FR are recorded in association with both LVF and HYP ictal onsets (Figures 12, 13) (Bragin et al.,1999b). FR-generating neuronal populations are not homogeneously distributed throughout the epileptogenic region, but exist in small neuronal clusters imbedded in more normal neuronal tissue (Figure 14) (Bragin et al., 2002). Both in vivo and in vitro studies have shown that the size of these FR-generating neuronal clusters can be increased by applying small amounts of bicuculline, a GABA antagonist (Figure 15) (Bragin et al., 2002). This suggests a possible mechanism of seizure generation in which small localized reductions in inhibition can permit FR-generating neuronal clusters to increase in size, coalesce, and ultimately give rise to widely dispersed hypersynchronous discharges (Engel et al., 2003). In this situation, the small localised reduction in inhibition ultimately results in initiation of a HYP ictal event that involves increased inhibition as well as increased excitation, underlying the fact that the role of

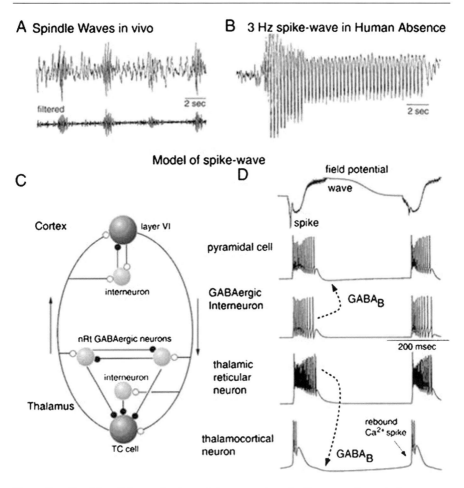

Figure 7.   Possible cellular mechanisms of the generation of spike-wave seizures in human absence. (A) Spindle waves during slow-wave sleep in the normal EEG are intermixed with delta waves and recur once every few seconds. (B) Single EEG trace during an absence attack illustrating the striking 3-Hz spike-wave activity that characterizes this state. This spike-wave activity is widely synchronised throughout the EEG (not shown). (C) Simplified diagram of thalamocortical interactions proposed to underlie the generation of some forms of spike-wave activities. Cortical pyramidal cells (in layer VI) and thalamocortical cells (TC cell) form mutually excitatory connections (open circles) that are regulated through the activation of GABAergic interneurons within the thalamus and cortex and thalamic reticular nucleus (nRt) (inhibitory synaptic connections are denoted with filled circles). (D) Simulation of one cycle of a spike-wave seizure in corticothalamic networks. A burst of spikes in a thalamocortical neuron activates the cortical network, which generates a strong burst of action potentials through intracortical recurrent excitatory connections. This activity strongly activates both local GABAergic neurons and thalamic reticular neurons. The buildup of K+ currents, including the activation of GABAB receptors and the inactivation of the depolarizing currents such as the low-threshold Ca2+ spike in thalamocortical cells, results in the cessation of activity in the network. The generation of a rebound Ca2+ spike in the thalamocortical cell, 300 ms later, initiates the next cycle of the oscillation. From McCormick and Contreras, 2001, with permission.

inhibition in ictogenesis is likely to be a complicated one involving both increases and decreases of specific inhibitory influences at different times and in different parts of the initiating structure, and even different parts of the neuron.

The preceding discussion is an over-simplification of a highly complex field of investigation that so far has elucidated potential mechanisms of seizure initiation in only a few of the recognised seizure types that occur in human epilepsy. There are, for instance, no animal models, and therefore no detailed invasive investigations on mechanisms of seizure initiation for myoclonic seizures, atonic seizures, or epileptic spasms, to name just a few of the ictal events responsible for severe disability associated with epilepsy.

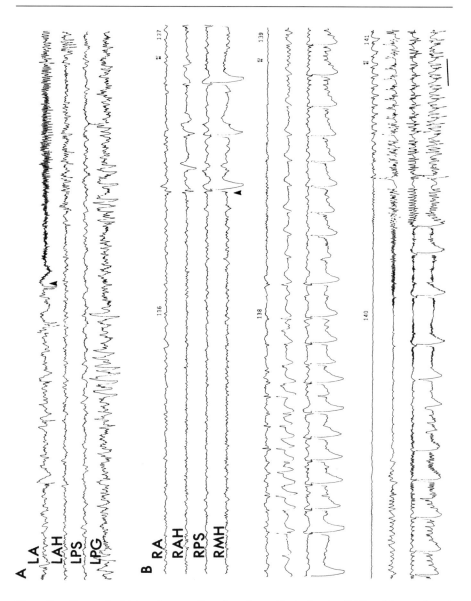

Figure 8. Segments of telemetry recordings from two patients showing EEG activity at selected depth electrode bipolar tips during the onset of complex partial seizures. A: The classic, depth electrode-recorded ictal onset consists of a buildup of low-voltage fast discharge, here beginning in a single channel (arrow). B: Three continuous segments show a more common ictal onset pattern, beginning with rhythmic, high-amplitude, sharp and slow transients (arrow), eventually giving way to a low-voltage fast discharge, which then evolves into higher-amplitude repetitive spikes or spikes-and-waves. L, left; R, right; A, amygdala; AH, anterior hippocampus; MH, midhippocampus; PS, presubiculum; PG, posterior hippocampal gyrus. Calibration 1 second. From Engel, 1988, with permission.

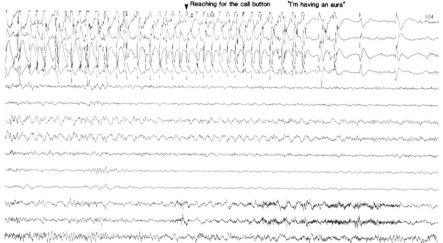

Figure 9.   Forty continuous seconds of an EEG recorded from depth, sphenoidal and scalp electrodes during a simple partial seizure of the right temporal lobe. Ictal onset consists of an increase in interictal spike discharges, maximal at the right anterior hippocampal electrode (left portion of upper panel). After 8-9 seconds, these spikes become regular, eventually developing into a 3-Hz spike-and-wave pattern involving all derivations from the right mesial temporal lobe. Note that no low-voltage fast activity is seen, either initially or at any part of the ictal episode. The patient reached for the call button at the arrow, at which point regular slow activity is also seen in the left anterior hippocampus and in the right sphenoidal electrode. The patient then indicated an aura consisting of a sensation of fear in her stomach. Depth electrode locations indicated as in Figure 8. Superficial contacts from anterior (A), mid (M), and posterior (P) depth electrodes recorded from cortex of middle temporal gyrus (MTG). Calibration 1 second. From Engel, 1988, with permission.

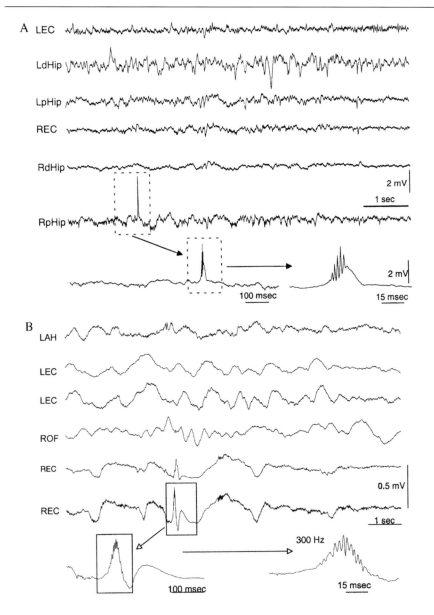

Figure 10. A: Example of KA-rat EEG with interictal spike with superimposed fast ripples. Abbreviations: LEC and REC left and right entorhinal cortex; LdHip and RdHip left and right dorsal hippocampus; LpHip and RpHip left and right posterior hippocampus. B: Interictal spike with superimposed fast ripples in the entorhinal cortex of a patient with mesial temporal lobe epilepsy. Arrows indicate extension of electrical activity indicated in the box. Abbreviations: LAH – left anterior hippocampus; ROF – right orbitofrontal cortex; LEC and REC – left and right entorhinal cortex (two microelectrodes in each side). From Bragin *et al.*, 1999a, with permission.

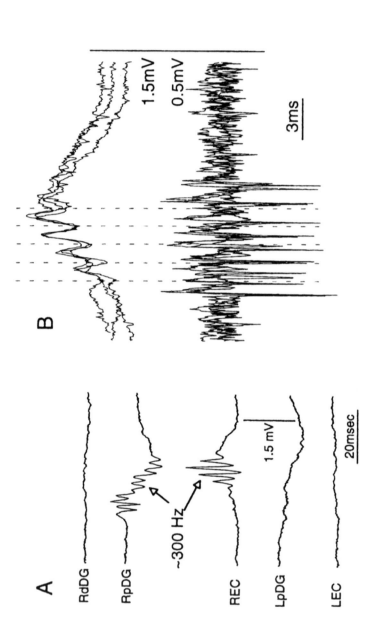

Figure 11. Fast ripples in the chronic epileptic rat brain. A: Spontaneous fast ripples recorded in the rat's dentate gyrus (DG) and EC 8 months after unilateral intrahippocampal KA injection. The recordings were performed in the right dorsal hippocampus and at symmetrical points in the right and left EC and ventral hippocampi. Notice that 300 Hz fast ripples occurs in the right ventral DG and ipsilateral EC. B: The unit activity of presumed pyramidal neurons (bottom) discharge in a phase locked fashion with the negative wave of the fast ripple. Three superimposed events are shown. This neuron revealed rare (less than 1 per 10 seconds) burst discharges with 1.5-2.0 msec interspike intervals. The fast ripples were recorded with 100-800 Hz band pass filter, unit activity was recorded with 0.5-5.0 kHz band pass filter. From Bragin *et al.*, 1999a, with permission.

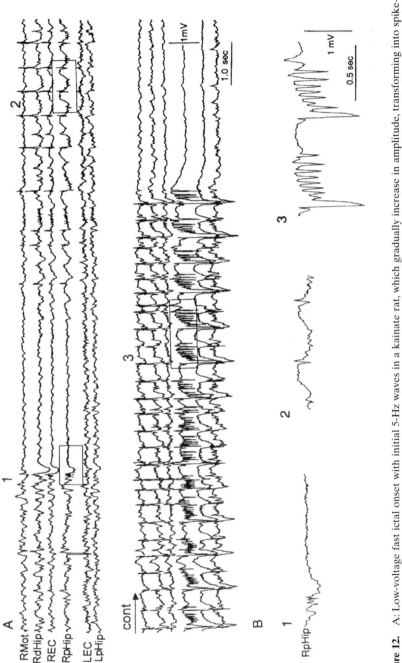

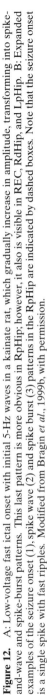

Figure 12. A: Low-voltage fast ictal onset with initial 5-Hz waves in a kainate rat, which gradually increase in amplitude, transforming into spike-and-wave and spike-burst patterns. This last pattern is more obvious in RpHip; however, it also is visible in REC, RdHip, and LpHip. B: Expanded examples of the seizure onset (1), spike wave (2) and spike burst (3) patterns in the RpHip are indicated by dashed boxes. Note that the seizure onset is a single spike with fast ripples. Modified from Bragin et al., 1999b, with permission.

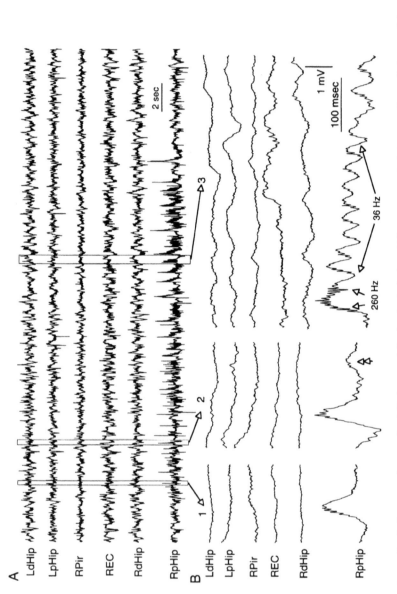
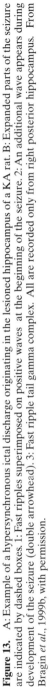

Figure 13. A: Example of a hypersynchronous ictal discharge originating in the lesioned hippocampus of a KA rat. B: Expanded parts of the seizure are indicated by dashed boxes. 1: Fast ripples superimposed on positive waves at the beginning of the seizure. 2: An additional wave appears during development of the seizure (double arrowhead). 3: Fast ripple tail gamma complex. All are recorded only from right posterior hippocampus. From Bragin *et al.*, 1999b, with permission.

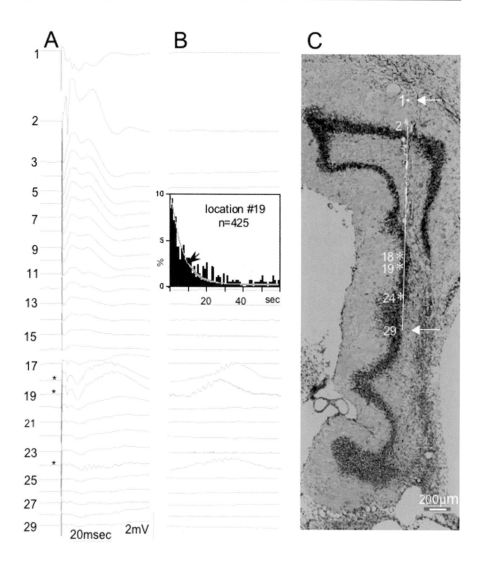

Figure 14. A, Voltage-depth profiles of potentials recorded at 100 μm intervals in response to perforant path stimulation. Note that FRs are evoked only at sites 18, 19, and 24. Recordings are averages of five stimulations at each site. B, Spontaneous FRs could be recorded only at the same sites as in A: 18, 19, and 24 (average of 5 in each trial). Inset illustrates distribution of spontaneous FRs (n = 425 FR events) recorded at location 19 during a period of 120 min. Arrow indicates mean inter-FR interval. C, Track of the microelectrode in a Nissl-stained coronal section of the posterior curve of the hippocampus, showing the dorsoventral extent of the dentate gyrus. Arrows indicate the beginning and the end of the recording area. Stars indicate sites at which FRs were recorded. Scale bar: gray, 200 μm on the basis of histological measurement; white, 200 μm on the basis of electrophysiological measurement. From Bragin *et al.*, 2002, with permission.

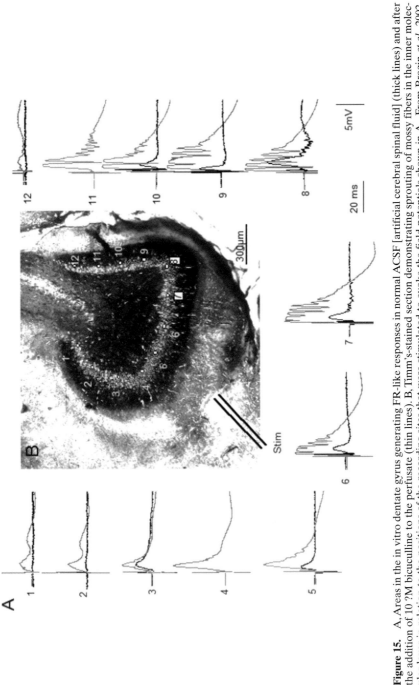
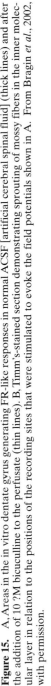

Figure 15. A, Areas in the in vitro dentate gyrus generating FR-like responses in normal ACSF [artificial cerebral spinal fluid] (thick lines) and after the addition of 10 ?M bicuculline to the perfusate (thin lines). B, Timm's-stained section demonstrating sprouting of mossy fibers in the inner molecular layer in relation to the positions of the recording sites that were stimulated to evoke the field potentials shown in A. From Bragin et al., 2002, with permission.

TURNING SEIZURES OFF

Recognising the fact that we still know very little about the fundamental mechanisms responsible for the actual initiation of epileptic seizures, as discussed in the previous section, even less is understood about fundamental mechanisms that cause epileptic seizures to stop (Engel *et al.*, 1997). What is clear, however, is that just as there are multiple types of seizure initiation, each reflecting one or more underlying neuronal mechanisms, there are also multiple types of seizure termination which must require distinctly different underlying neuronal mechanisms.

Generalised tonic-clonic seizures consist of a tonic phase which evolves into a clonic phase characterised by EEG discharges separated by periods of EEG depression. Often, the discharges become further and further apart and eventually disappear, leaving the EEG depressed for a variable duration during the postictal state. This is not an invariable pattern of termination for these ictal events; at times the electrographic ictal discharge does not include a clear clonic phase and gradually deteriorates, with no specific point on the EEG at which the ictal event ends and the postictal period begins (Figure 5). Many LVF focal seizures show similar EEG patterns of termination and focal EEG depression during the postictal period. Whereas consciousness returns gradually after most generalised tonic-clonic seizures, representing residual global cerebral dysfunction, focal seizures may be followed by varying periods of focal neurological disturbances, the classical example being Todd's paresis of the body part involved in the focal-motor seizure.

Generalised and focal LVF ictal events are believed to be terminated by the phasing in of active inhibitory processes, as well as depolarisation block, electrogenic pumps, and changes in the ionic environment, which then produce the postictal signs and symptoms. Both animal and human studies suggest that the active inhibitory mechanisms engaged to terminate seizures not only involve the inhibitory neurotransmitter GABA, but also other neurotransmitters and neuromodulators such as adenosine and opioid peptides (Engel *et al.*, 1997). More information about natural homeostatic mechanisms that are responsible for ictal termination may aid in the development of novel approaches for controlling epileptic seizures; however, it is also possible that at least some of these mechanisms are associated with neuronal disturbances that contribute not only to postictal, but also interictal, cerebral dysfunction. Approaches to enhancing these mechanisms, therefore, could result in an increased incidence of interictal behavioral disturbances.

Typical absence seizures end abruptly with no postictal EEG or behavioral abnormalities (Figure 6) (Engel *et al.*, 1997). This suggests that neuronal mechanisms of seizure termination for HYP ictal events are not the same as those discussed for generalised tonic-clonic seizures, but, rather, involve a desynchronising influence, which has no subsequent EEG or behavioral consequence. Paradoxically, however, benzodiazepines, which facilitate GABA-mediated inhibition, can terminate absences seizures, indicating that active inhibition, perhaps acting on the pacemaker influence of the nucleus reticularis (Figure 7), may also play a role in absence seizure termination, again underlying the complicated role of inhibition as both pro- and anti-epileptogenic.

Focal HYP seizures in mesial temporal structures also end abruptly, without postictal EEG depression, suggesting neuronal mechanisms of termination more similar to those of absence seizures than to those of focal LVF ictal events. Inadequate data are available to suggest what these neuronal mechanisms of seizure termination might be, or why these events often are transformed into focal LVF seizures.

As with ictal initiation, there are no detailed invasive investigations on seizure termination for many seizure types, including myoclonic seizures, atonic seizures, and epileptic spasms. It is likely that some or all of these unique ictal events involve the engagement of unique seizure-suppressing mechanisms that cause them to be self-limited, and that are distinctly different from those discussed in the previous paragraphs.

Continuous seizures, or status epilepticus, result from failure of natural seizure-terminating mechanisms (Wasterlain and Treiman, 2006). Generalised convulsive status epilepticus is a life-threatening condition, but absence status also occurs and can be severely disabling. Focal motor status epilepticus is referred to as epilepsia partialis continua of Kojevnikov, and focal non-motor status is referred to as aura continua. These events, which can persist for days or even months, are of particular interest because they indicate that mechanisms which limit the spread of epileptic discharges in the brain are independent of those mechanisms which terminate ictal events. It is likely, therefore, that any given seizure gives rise to multiple homeostatic neuronal mechanisms that act to suppress various aspects of the ictal event, and that failure of some of these protective mechanisms determines how seizures evolve, while failure of others determines how long they last. It is also important to recognise that at least some of these homeostatic mechanisms also disrupt normal cerebral function, which in some cases can be as, or even more, disabling than the seizures themselves. Understanding the fundamental neuronal basis of these natural protective reactions to epileptic seizures could lead to effective interventions to prevent or reverse disabling interictal behavioural disturbances.

CONCLUSIONS

There are many types of epileptic seizures, and many reasons for their occurrence. Consequently, there is no single pathophysiological mechanism responsible for seizure generation, or for seizure termination. Because there are clinical opportunities for invasive research and/or animal models for some types of focal seizures, as well as generalised tonic-clonic and typical absence seizures, specific alterations in the balance of excitatory and inhibitory neuronal influences, and abnormal hyper-synchronisation, have been identified as mechanisms for seizure initiation. Little is known, however, about mechanisms that initiate many other ictal events, such as myoclonic and atonic seizures or epileptic spasms, where clinical investigations are more difficult and adequate animal models do not exist. Generalised tonic-clonic and many focal seizures can be terminated by various mechanisms, including active inhibitory processes, depolarisation block, electrogenic pumps, and changes in the ionic environment, which are then responsible for postictal signs and symptoms. Other mechanisms must be responsible for terminating hyper-synchronous ictal events, such as absence seizures, however, because there are no postictal disturbances. Most ictal events are not the result of a single pathophysiological process, but an evolution involving progression from one epileptogenic process to another, with specific homeostatic mechanisms that can abort progression; failure of these mechanisms results in various forms of status epilepticus, which can continue as one part of the seizure without evolving to another, as in epilepsia partialis continua. Much more research is necessary to elucidate the pathophysiological mechanisms that turn all seizures on and off.

ACKNOWLEDGEMENTS

Original research reported by the author was supported in part by Grants NS-02808, NS-15654, NS-33310, and NS-42372 from the National Institutes of Health.

REFERENCES

Babb, T.L. and Crandall, P.H. (1976). Epileptogenesis of human limbic neurons in psychomotor epileptics. *Electroencephalogr Clin Neurophysiol* **40**, 225-243.

Bragin, A., Engel, J. Jr., Wilson, C.L., Fried, I. and Mathern, G.W. (1999a). Hippocampal and entorhinal cortex high frequency oscillations (100-500 Hz) in kainic acid-treated rats with chronic seizures and human epileptic brain. *Epilepsia* **40**, 127-137.

Bragin, A., Engel, J. Jr., Wilson, C.L., Vizentin, E. and Mathern, G.W. (1999b). Electrophysiologic analysis of a chronic seizure model after unilateral hippocampal KA injection. *Epilepsia* **40**, 1210-1221.

Bragin, A., Mody, I., Wilson, C.L. and Engel, J. Jr. (2002). Local generation of fast ripples in epileptic brain. *J Neurosci* **22**, 2012-2021.

Commission on Classification and Terminology of the International League Against Epilepsy. Proposal for revised clinical and electroencephalographic classification of epileptic seizures (1981). *Epilepsia* **22**, 489-501.

Engel, J. Jr. (1988). Brain metabolism and pathophysiology of human epilepsy. In: Dichter, M. (Ed), *Mechanisms of Epileptogenesis: Transition to Seizure*. Plenum Press, New York, pp.1-15.

Engel J Jr. (1989). *Seizures and Epilepsy*. F. A. Davis, Philadelphia.

Engel, J. Jr. (1990). Functional explorations of the human epileptic brain and their therapeutic implications. *Electroencephalogr Clin Neurophysiol* **76**, 296-316.

Engel J Jr. (2001) A proposed diagnostic scheme for people with epileptic seizures and with epilepsy. Report of the ILAE Task Force on Classification and Terminology. *Epilepsia* **42**, 796-803.

Engel, J. Jr., Lubens, P., Kuhl, D.E. and Phelps M. (1985). Local cerebral metabolic rate for glucose during petit mal absences. *Ann Neurol* **17**, 121-128.

Engel, J. Jr., Dichter, M. and Schwartzkroin, P. (1997). Basic mechanisms of human epilepsy. In: Engel, J. Jr. and Pedley, T.A. (Eds), *Epilepsy: A Comprehensive Textbook*. Lippincott-Raven, Philadelphia, pp.499-512.

Engel, J. Jr., Wilson, C. and Bragin, A. (2003). Advances in understanding the process of epileptogenesis based on patient material: What can the patient tell us? *Epilepsia* **44** (Suppl. 12), S60-S71.

Fisher, R.S., van Emde Boas, W., Blume, W., Elger, C., Engel, J. Jr., Genton, P. and Lee, P. (2005). Epileptic seizures and epilepsy. Definitions proposed by the International League against Epilepsy (ILAE) and the International Bureau for Epilepsy (IBE). *Epilepsia* **46**, 470-472.

Giaretta, D., Avoli, M. and Gloor, P. (1987). Intracellular recordings in pericruciate neurons during spike and wave discharges of feline generalized penicillin epilepsy. *Brain Res* **405**, 68-79.

Matsumoto, H. and Ajmone-Marsan, C. (1964a). Cortical cellular phenomena in experimental epilepsy: Interictal manifestations. *Exp Neurol* **9**, 286-304.

Matsumoto, H. and Ajmone-Marsan, C. (1964b). Cortical cellular phenomena in experimental epilepsy: Ictal manifestations. *Exp Neurol* **9**, 305-326.

McCormick, D.A. and Contreras, D. (2001). On the cellular and network bases of epileptic seizures. *Ann Rev Physiol* **63**, 815-846.

Wasterlain, C.G. and Treiman, D.M. (Eds), (2006). *Status Epilepticus: Mechanisms and Management.* MIT Press, Boston (in press).

Seizure Freedom: Clinical, Research and Quality of Life Perspectives
Edited by Michael R. Trimble
© 2006 Clarius Press Ltd

4

Rational Polypharmacy: Which Combinations are Most Likely to Lead to Seizure Freedom?

MATTHEW C. WALKER

*Department of Clinical and Experimental Epilepsy,
Institute of Neurology, UCL,
London, UK*

INTRODUCTION

The concept of combining drugs in order to improve efficacy is not new, and has met with considerable success in other therapeutic areas such as antibiotics and cancer chemotherapy. In epilepsy, combined tablets have been available, most notably phelantin – a combination of phenytoin, phenobarbital and metamphetamine (Davidson and Berman, 1956). This approach of a combination pill has been abandoned due to the individual titration of each drug that is usually necessary. Nevertheless, the approach of combining drugs offers the possibility of improved efficacy, but this may be at the expense of increased side-effects, drug interactions, difficulties with compliance and greater complexity of management.

A combination of anti-epileptic drugs (AEDs) can result in improved efficacy in three different ways. The combination could be supra-additive (i.e. the efficacy of the combination is greater than the combination of the efficacies), additive or infra-additive (i.e. the efficacy of the combination is less that the combination of the efficacies). Although both theoretical and experimental studies have added to our understanding of the additive effects of combination therapies, the categorisation of combination therapies as supra- or infra-additive is not the sole consideration. Most AED doses are restricted by side-effects (Mattson *et al.*, 1985). If it is possible to have an increase in efficacy with fewer side-effects than would be expected by increasing the dose of one of the components, then this is a useful outcome. There is unfortunately a poverty of well-designed clinical trials addressing the benefits of polytherapy against monotherapy, and therefore much of the rational for polytherapy is informed by theoretical considerations and animal data. Here I will first review the rationale based upon mode of action and specific problems with this approach, secondly I will review the animal evidence for combination therapy and lastly the human evidence.

MODE OF ACTION OF ANTI-EPILEPTIC DRUGS

If two drugs have exactly the same target, then the combination is likely to be infra-additive, as each drug will compete for the same target. Thus drugs acting on different targets are more likely to be supra-additive (synergistic). This is especially so if a particular process depends on more than one pathway, so that inhibition of one pathway can be compensated by another. An example of this is GABA uptake, as there are a group of GABA transporters (GAT1, GAT2, GAT3) (Borden, 1996). Inhibition of GAT1 or GAT2/3 results in a small increase in extracellular GABA because the uninhibited GAT compensates, so preventing a large rise in extracellular GABA (Keros and Hablitz, 2005). Inhibition of both GAT1 and GAT2/3, however, prevents compensation from occurring and so results in a large rise in extracellular GABA (Keros and Hablitz, 2005).

This concept comprises one of the main theoretical approaches to combination therapy (the combination of drugs with different targets is likely to be more effective than combining drugs with the same targets). However, the same target is not equivalent to the same class of AED. Drugs that belong to one class of drugs (e.g. those that act on the GABAergic system) can have very different actions and could be supra-additive (see below) or could act on similar, but distinct targets, as has been demonstrated above in which two GABA transporter inhibitors acting on different GABA transporters are synergistic. Further, although it is appealing to identify a single target for each AED, this belies the intricacies of AED mechanisms of action. Most AEDs drugs have a number of putative targets (frequently these have been only partially determined), and it is often not entirely clear which is the most relevant for the drug's anti-epileptic action. There can also be complex consequences, even when an AED has only one putative target (e.g. tiagabine inhibiting GAT1). Most of the AEDs that we use are commonly divided into three classes: drugs that act on sodium channels, calcium channels or the GABAergic system.

Sodium channels

Voltage-gated sodium channels are responsible for the rising phase of the action potential in excitable cells and membranes, and are thus critical for action potential generation and propagation. The sodium channel exists in three principal conformational states:

    a. at hyperpolarised potentials the channel is in the resting closed state;

    b. with depolarisation the channels convert to an open state that conducts sodium ions;

    c. the channel then enters a closed, non-conducting, inactivated state (Catterall, 1999).

Many drugs including certain anaesthetics and anti-arrhythmic agents exert their therapeutic effect by preferential binding to the inactivated state of the sodium channel (Catterall, 2000a). This has two effects: first to shift the voltage dependence of inactivation towards the resting potential (i.e the channels become inactive at lower membrane potentials), and secondly to delay the return of the channel to the resting, closed confirmation following hyperpolarisation. Phenytoin, lamotrigine and carbamazepine have a similar mode of action. All bind in the inner pore of the sodium channel, and their binding is mutually exclusive (Kuo, 1998). There may, however, be differences in the fashion in which each of these drugs interacts with adjacent amino acids that may partly explain drug specific effects. How does this binding mediate their anticonvulsant effect? The conventional view has been that such binding prevents sustained repetitive firing. The rate at which an axon can 'fire' is critically determined by the rate at which the sodium channels change from the inactivated state to the resting, active state ready to be reactivated by a subsequent depolarisation (Catterall, 2000a). If this time is delayed, then the 'refractory period' is prolonged. Thus phenytoin, carbamazepine, lamotrigine and oxcarbazepine all prolong the 'refractory period' and so inhibit sustained repetitive firing. In addition, since these drugs bind to channels in their inactive state, then the greater the number of channels that have entered this state, the greater the drug binding. This results in a 'use dependent' phenomenon in which repetitive firing results in greater amounts of the drug bound and so greater inhibition. Since lamotrigine, carbamazepine and phenytoin act at the same site in similar fashions, then if the epilepsy is resistant to one will it be resistant to the others? This does not seem to be the case; a sodium channel may be resistant to carbamazepine, but respond in a normal manner to lamotrigine and phenytoin (Remy and Beck, 2006).

It has been argued that since these drugs have similar modes of action then combinations of these drugs offer no benefit beyond that of using higher concentrations of one. Indeed, the combinations would be expected to be infra-additive, as there would be competition for the same target. This, however, does not comprise the only clinical consideration. Often the dose of AED is limited by side-effects. Some of these side-effects may be independent of these drugs' action at sodium channels. So that if an epilepsy partially responds to one of these drugs, but further increases in dose are limited by side-effects, then the addition of a drug that acts at the same site, but has a different spectrum of side-effects may have an additional benefit.

Do other AEDs have similar effects on the sodium channel? Oxcarbazepine is likely to have a similar effect to carbamazepine (Mclean *et al.*, 1994). Valproate seems to inhibit rapid repetitive firing (Mclean and Macdonald, 1986), but acts at a different site from the site on which carbamazepine, lamotrigine and phenytoin act. The new AEDs topiramate and zonisamide, may also have an action on sodium channels, the exact nature of which is unclear (White, 1999). Thus from a theoretical perspective, it is unclear whether these drugs will compete with the actions of carbamazepine, lamotrigine and phenytoin. Indeed an action on sodium channel at a different site could have a synergistic effect.

Calcium channels

In brain, there are 4 main classes of voltage gated calcium channel expressed, L, P/Q, N and T type channels(Catterall, 2000b). L, P/Q and N type channels require large depolarisations before opening, whilst the T type channel is activated at relatively hyperpolarised potentials, and only requires small depolarisation in order to open. All but the L-type calcium channel open transiently before rapidly inactivating. The L-type channel opens for longer resulting in sustained calcium entry. Each of the channels has a different cellular and brain distribution, and thus drugs that act at different calcium channels are likely to have very different effects, and so could theoretically compliment one another. Of note is that drugs ostensibly from the same class (e.g. sodium channel antagonists) can have actions at very different calcium channels.

T-type channels play an integral role in the generation of spike-wave discharges of absence seizures (McCormick and Contreras, 2001). Ethosuximide, an effective anti-absence drug, has been proposed to inhibit specifically T-type calcium channels (Coulter *et al.*, 1989). Furthermore, other drugs (e.g. zonisamide, valproate) that are effective in absence seizures have also been proposed to act at T-type calcium channels. There are thus theoretical reasons to suspect that these drugs may be infra-additive. However, even the archetypal drug in this class, ethosuximide, has other effects that may contribute to its anti-epileptic action such as actions on persistent sodium currents and calcium-dependent potassium currents (Leresche *et al.*, 1998).

The GABAergic system

Gamma-amino-butyric acid (GABA) is the major inhibitory neurotransmitter in the brain. It is formed and degraded in the GABA shunt. Glutamic acid decarboxylase (GAD) converts glutamate to GABA. GABA is degraded by GABA transaminase to succinic semialdehyde; alpha-ketoglutarate accepts the amino group in this reaction to become glutamate. GABA acts at three specific receptor types: $GABA_A$, $GABA_B$ and $GABA_C$ receptors. $GABA_C$ receptors are present almost exclusively within the retina. GABA is taken up from the extracellular space by GABA transporters. Thus, to state that a drug 'works on the GABAergic system' is a vast over-simplification. The present 'GABAergic' AEDs that we use prevent GABA uptake (tiagabine), prevent GABA breakdown (vigabatrin), or act on $GABA_A$ receptors (e.g. barbiturate, benzodiazepines) (Czuczwar and Patsalos, 2001). They, therefore, have different targets. Even when there seems to be one target (e.g. $GABA_A$ receptors) there is essentially more than one target. Indeed the diversity of $GABA_A$ receptors is a good example of how a rational approach based on drug mechanisms is fraught with difficulties.

$GABA_A$ receptors are mainly expressed post-synaptically within the brain. $GABA_A$ receptors are constructed from five of at least 16 mammalian subunits, grouped in seven classes: α, β, γ, δ, σ, ϵ and π (Mehta and Ticku, 1999). This permits a vast number of putative receptor isoforms. The subunit composition determines the specific effects of allosteric modulators of $GABA_A$ receptors, such as neurosteroids, zinc and benzodiazepines (Mehta and Ticku, 1999). The subunit composition also determines the kinetics of the receptors and can affect desensitisation. Importantly the subunit composition of $GABA_A$ receptors expressed in neurons can change during epileptogenesis, and these changes influence the pharmacodynamic response to drugs (Brooks-Kayal et al., 1998). $GABA_A$ receptor activation results in the early rapid component of inhibitory transmission. $GABA_A$ receptor activation conventionally results in an influx of chloride and cellular hyperpolarisation.

Benzodiazepines are specific modulators of $GABA_A$ receptors and act at $GABA_A$ receptors that contain a $\alpha1$, $\alpha2$, $\alpha3$ or $\alpha5$ subunit in combination with a γ subunit. Drugs acting at the benzodiazepine site have different affinities for the different α subunit containing $GABA_A$ receptors, and this specificity can affect pharmacodynamic response. This is due perhaps to the varied distribution of these receptors in the brain. Thus the $\alpha1$ subunit containing receptors seem to have mainly a sedative effect, and are perhaps responsible for this side-effect of benzodiazepines (Rudolph and Mohler, 2006). This may also explain why zolpidem, a drug that has greater affinity for $GABA_A$ receptors containing the $\alpha1$ subunit has marked sedative effects and weak anticonvulsant efficacy. More selective ligands could thus result in benzodiazepine agonists that have less sedative effect and greater anticonvulsant potential. The benzodiazepines main effect is to increase the affinity of $GABA_A$ receptors for GABA, and to prolong receptor opening times.

Barbiturates are less selective than benzodiazepines, and potentiate $GABA_A$ receptor mediated currents. In addition, at high concentrations, they can directly activate the $GABA_A$ receptor. This may partly explain their anaesthetic effect at high concentrations. Other anaesthetic agents, such as propofol, have similar effects on the $GABA_A$ receptors.

Topiramate can also potentiate $GABA_A$ receptors, but more specifically those containing $\alpha4$ subunits (Cipelletti et al., 2002). These receptors are high affinity, extrasynaptic receptors that may mediate a tonically active $GABA_A$ receptor mediated current (Semyanov et al., 2004). $GABA_A$ receptors have other modulatory sites, and can be modulated by zinc and neurosteroids. Neurosteroids are of interest as they act on δ subunit containing GABAA receptors, and variations in neurosteroid levels may explain why seizures occasionally cluster around the time of menstruation (Maguire et al., 2005).

$GABA_A$ receptor agonists can also exacerbate absence seizures. Absence seizures are generated within a recurrent loop between the thalamus and neocortex, and their generation is dependent upon oscillatory behaviour mediated by $GABA_A$ receptors, $GABA_B$ receptors, T type calcium channels, the cationic conductance Ih and glutamate receptors (McCormick and Contreras, 2001). One hypothesis is that hyperpolarisation of the thalamocortical neurons in the thalamus mediated by GABAergic inhibition leads to activation of Ih and T type calcium currents resulting in neuronal depolarisation and spikes that activate neurons in the neocortex, which in turn stimulate the thalamic reticular nucleus, leading to GABAergic inhibition of the thalamocortical neurons, and so the cycle continues. Non-specific $GABA_A$ receptor agonists, $GABA_B$ receptor agonists or agonists of specific $GABA_A$ receptors can all hyperpolarise thalamocortical neurons and so can have a pro-absence effect. This occurs with GABA uptake inhibitors, which may thus antagonise the actions of anti-absence medication.

Other means of modulating GABAergic activity are to inhibit GABA uptake or GABA breakdown. GABA is mainly metabolised by GABA transaminase to succinic semialdehyde; glutamate is synthesised in this reaction (see above). Vigabatrin irreversibly inhibits GABA transaminase. This results in an increase in intracellular GABA that can produce an increase in vesicular GABA, and so inhibitory transmission. In addition, vigabatrin results in an increase in extracellular GABA that may be partly due to decreased GABA uptake (Wu et al., 2003). GABA released into the extracellular space is transported into neurones and glial cells via Na^+/Cl^- coupled GABA transporters (GAT) that can transport GABA against an osmotic gradient (Borden, 1996). In human and rat, four GAT proteins have been identified and cloned: GAT-1, GAT-2, GAT-3 and BGT-1 (Borden, 1996). These transporters have different regional and interregional localisations. GAT-1 is predominantly present on pre-synaptic GABAeregic terminals and glia, and is the most prevalent GABA transporter in the rat forebrain. In contrast, GAT-3 is localised exclusively to astrocytes and glia, and GAT-2 has a more diffuse distribution.

Tiagabine is a GAT-1 specific, non-transportable, lipid soluble GABA uptake inhibitor, and as has previously been discussed, combinations of tiagabine with GAT-2/3 inhibitors have a supra-additive effect on extracellular GABA (Keros and Hablitz, 2005); thus drugs acting on similar, but not identical targets can be supra-additive. Tiagabine in contrast to vigabatrin has no effect on total brain GABA (Sills *et al.*, 1999). The combination of a drug that increases total brain GABA and one that increases the extracellular GABA concentration may be supra-additive, and such a supra-additive effect of vigabatrin and tiagabine has been noted in brain slice experiments (Kohling *et al.*, 2002).

Vigabatrin and tiagabine serve as further examples of how we incompletely understand drug mechanisms of action. Although many explanations of the mode of action of vigabatrin and tiagabine concentrate on raising the extracellular GABA concentration, these drugs may have two other critical effects. The time-course of the GABA transient in the synaptic cleft is partly (and variably) determined by GABA uptake; tiagabine can thus prolong the synaptic GABA transient (Nusser *et al.*, 2001). In addition, by decreasing GABA uptake there is greater spill-over of GABA from the synaptic cleft onto extra-synaptic receptors (Overstreet and Westbrook, 2003). This results in an effect that is similar to, although mechanistically different from the effect of benzodiazepines and barbiturates – an effect that may be potentiated by these drugs. This raises the possibility that these drugs could act synergistically.

Furthermore, increasing extracellular GABA can have two opposing effects: it can increase the activation of extrasynaptic receptors and can thus enhance the tonic current (Semyanov *et al.*, 2004). A second effect of increasing extracellular GABA is to desensitise synaptic $GABA_A$ receptors (Overstreet and Westbrook, 2001). This can result in smaller amplitude $GABA_A$ receptor mediated currents. Thus vigabatrin increases tonic inhibition, but decreases synaptically mediated inhibition (Overstreet and Westbrook, 2001).

Spill-over of neurotransmitter may enhance not only $GABA_A$ receptor mediated transmission, but also $GABA_B$ receptor mediated effects. Enhancement of $GABA_B$ receptor activation will not only have a post-synaptic effect, but also a pre-synaptic effect and will decrease the release of GABA from GABAergic terminals (decreasing inhibition), and glutamate from glutamatergic terminals (decreasing excitation). The overall effect on the network is thus difficult to predict.

Other mechanisms

Although the main classes of drug mechanisms are discussed above, many new AEDs have novel or multiple modes of action. Indeed, it is likely that even the older AEDs have multiple actions leading to dissimilarities between drugs that have been proposed to act on the same target. This can be seen with lamotrigine, which in contrast to phenytoin and carbamazepine, is effective in absence seizures (Buoni *et al.*, 1999). It seems, at first sight, paradoxical that three drugs that act on the same target should have opposing effects in absence seizures. Lamotrigine has recently been found to have a significant effect on a different channel, Ih, and its effect on this could explain the different spectrum of activity for this drug (Poolos *et al.*, 2002).

The newer AEDs gabapentin and pregabalin may have an effect on presynaptic calcium channels (Sills, 2006). These drugs are effective in partial epilepsy and their novel mode of action suggests that they could be synergistic with antiepileptic drugs in partial epilepsy. Zonisamide, topiramate and levetiracetam have broad spectrums of activity and novel modes of action. The main mode of action of topiramate is still unclear, although actions have been proposed at $GABA_A$ receptors, sodium channels and glutamate receptors (White, 1999). Similarly the main mode of action of zonisamide is unclear. Levetiracetam has been found to bind to the synaptic vesicular protein, SV2A, although how this mediates its anti-epileptic effect is unknown (Lynch *et al.*, 2004). These latter drugs with distinct, novel modes of actions are thus more likely to demonstrate synergistic effects with other AEDs in both partial and generalised epilepsies.

This analysis of mechanisms of actions above hopefully serves to illustrate the complexity of the situation. Certain combinations are more likely to demonstrate synergism, especially combining AEDs with new AEDs that have unique mechanisms of action or combining drugs with different mechanisms of action. Nevertheless, the results of combining drugs within the same class (e.g. GABAergic drugs) are difficult to predict and many may show synergism. Perhaps, the most robust conclusion is that combining phenytoin, carbamazepine or lamotrigine is likely to have an infra-additive effect. Similarly, combining valproate and ethosuximide in absences may also be infra-additive.

ANIMAL EVIDENCE FOR DRUG COMBINATIONS

There may be theoretical reasons to suspect synergistic or infra-additive effects, but the most direct test would be to assess this in vivo in humans or in animal models. The assessment of drug combinations in animal models is, however, not straightforward and there are a number of potential pitfalls. Simply adding a sub-therapeutic dose of one drug to another and showing efficacy tells us nothing about the potency of a combination. This can be easily illustrated by the example of combining a drug with itself. The addition of sub-therapeutic doses of the same drug can result in a therapeutic dose. Thus more complex methods of combining drugs is needed. A standard method is the isobolic method (isobolographic analysis). In this analysis, two drugs (A and B) are compared. A specific efficacy endpoint (usually the dose that results in protection against seizures in 50% of animals – ED50) is chosen. Experiments are then carried out to determine the ED50 for each individual drug, and this gives the relative potencies for each drug. ED50s are then calculated for various combination ratios of A and B, and plotted on graph of the dose of drug A versus dose of drug B. If the drugs are additive then the ED50s for each drug will lie on a straight line joining the ED50 for A to the ED50 for B (see Figure 1). If the combination is supra-additive then the points will lie below this line, and if the drugs are infra-additive, then they will lie above this line (Figure 1).

An alternative approach is to use a seizure model that does not respond to one drug (A) at any dose, and then to see if combining this drug with another drug (B) affects the ED50 for drug B. These approaches have been used for a number of drug combinations and the results are summarised in Table 1. These results do not form an obvious pattern, except that sodium channel antagonists are often infra-additive. There are however a number of caveats concerning the clinical usefulness of these methods. The first is the choice of seizure model. Most of these studies have been carried out in models of acutely induced seizures that may not always be a good representative of spontaneously occurring seizures. Indeed, levetiracetam was shown to be ineffective in many of the standard acute seizure models, yet is an effective AED (Klitgaard, 2001).

Figure 1:   Isobolographic assessment of pharmacodynamic interaction. Points falling on the line indicate additive effects, points above are indicative of infra-additive effects, points below the line are indicative of supra-additive effects.

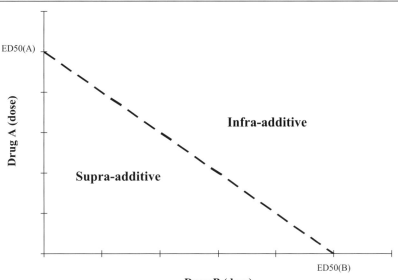

Table 1:   Efficacy of combinations in animal models

	CBZ	CLN	ESM	FBM	GBP	LMG	LEV	OXC	PB	DPH	TGB	TPM	VPA	VGB
Carbamazepine (CBZ)			–	+	–	+	0	0				+0		
Clonazepam (CLN)				0		+		+/–					0	
Ethosuximide (ESM)				0									0/–	
Felbamate (FBM)	–	0	0		0	0		–	+/0	–	0	+	0/–	
Gabapentin (GBP)	+		0			+		+	+	+	+	–	+	
Lamotrigine (LMG)	–	+	0	+			0	–	+		0	+	+	
Levetiracetam (LEV)	+				0			+	0	0		+	0	
Oxcarbazepine (OXC)	0	+/–	–	+	–	+			0	–	0	+	0	
Phenobarbitone (PB)	0			+/0	+	+	0	0		0/+		+	0	+
Phenytoin (DPH))				–	+		0	–	0/+			0	+	
Tiagabine (TGB)				0	+	0		0				0+		
Topiramate (TPM)	+			+	–	+	+	+	+	0	0		+	–
Valproate (VPA)	0		0/–	0/–	+	+	0	0	0	+	+	+		0
Vigabatrin (VGB)		0	+						+			–	0	

+ = supra-additive, 0 = additive, – = infra-additive.

Data taken from (Borowicz et al., 2002; 2004;   Bourgeois, 1986; 1988a; 1988b;   Bourgeois and Wad, 1988;   Luszczki and Czuczwar, 2003; 2004a; 2004b; 2005a; 2005b;   Luszczki et al., 2003a; 2003b; 2003c; 2003d; 2005a; 2005b; 2006;   Masuda et al., 1981;   Sills et al., 2004;   Van Rijn et al., 2004.)

Secondly, because efficacy is supra-additive in one model does not neces-sarily mean that it will be supra-additive in another model, again raising the question of the validity of extrapolating these results to humans. Furthermore, pharmacokinetic interactions have to be taken into considera-tion and not only peripheral pharmacokinetics but also brain penetration. Thus the demonstration of supra-additive efficacy may not be due to a pharmacodynamic effect but due to increased brain penetration of one of the drugs. Nevertheless, this may still be a useful clinical outcome (see below). Lastly in the clinical situation it is not just the efficacy of a drug that is of importance, but also the adverse effects. Even though a drug combination is additive or infra-additive if this results in a combination with fewer side-effects than higher doses of the single drugs, then this may be a clinically useful combination. Indeed, it is possible to investigate this using animal models by looking at both the efficacy of combinations against seizures and the toxicity of combinations. Thus valproate and ethosuximide in the pentylenetetrazol animal model were shown in one study to have additive efficacy, but infra-additive toxicity (Bourgeois, 1988b).

HUMAN EVIDENCE FOR DRUG COMBINATIONS

In the clinical arena, combination therapy (polytherapy) has a poor reputa-tion compared to monotherapy, for good reason. Polytherapy can result in drug interactions, poor compliance, and increased side-effects. Yet we may have been undervaluing polytherapy, as we have not been comparing like with like. Deckers and colleagues (1997) have pointed out that we should perhaps be considering drug load. In this analysis the drug load is the dose of a drug divided by the defined daily dose (assigned by the WHO). Thus a high dose of a drug in monotherapy may represent a higher drug load than a combination of drugs at low dose in polytherapy. Our method of instigating polytherapy necessarily increases drug load – we increase a drug in monotherapy to the maximum tolerated and then add other AEDs. Perhaps, we would think more favourably of polytherapy if we used the drugs at lower doses so not increasing the total drug load.

What is the clinical evidence for the benefits of drug combinations? Unfortunately, there are very few trials that specifically address this issue. Most trials of new AEDs involve adding the drug to an established drug regimen. Efficacy in such trials could be viewed as evidence of the value of combination therapy, but what is usually not clear is whether the additional effect is secondary to the added drug alone or its combination with other AEDs. Some randomised, double-blind, add-on trials of new AEDs in refrac-tory epilepsy have been followed by a withdrawal to a monotherapy trial.

Withdrawal of a drug can result in rebound seizures making it difficult to determine whether an increase in seizures is due to this or a lesser efficacy of the monotherapy compared to polytherapy.

Such studies have suggested that a substantial part of the benefit of add-on AEDs may be due to efficacy of the add-on drug alone rather than the combination of drugs. An exception to this is a study that was carried out with lamotrigine (Brodie and Yuen, 1997); this study was not, however, specifically designed to investigate the efficacy of combination therapy. Lamotrigine was added to carbamazepine, phenytoin or valproate monotherapy. Those who experienced at least a 50% reduction in seizures could have their original therapy tapered leaving them on lamotrigine monotherapy. During the conversion to monotherapy, the lamotrigine dose could be adjusted to compensate for a serum level rise (on removal of an enzyme inducing drug) that results in side-effects or a fall (removal of valproate) that results in loss of seizure control. Withdrawal to monotherapy from the combination with phenytoin or carbamazepine resulted in a decrease in seizures. The interpretation of this result is confounded by those who dropped out of the study and by a general increase in the lamotrigine serum levels. More interestingly, there was an increase in seizure frequency in those withdrawn to lamotrigine monotherapy from the combination with valproate despite an increase in the lamotrigine serum levels. This provides some evidence that the combination of valproate and lamotrigine may be of clinical benefit (so long as the combination does not result in an unacceptable increase in side-effects). This combination has gained further support from a study of valproate, lamotrigine or their combination as add-on. The combination resulted in responses when there had been non response to add-on of the individual drugs (Pisani *et al.*, 1999).

There have been other approaches to assessing the efficacy of combination therapy. These have been designed to address three questions:

1. Is combination therapy more effective than monotherapy when controlling for drug load?
2. Is combination therapy more effective than substitution of one monotherapy by another?
3. If monotherapy with two drugs has failed will combination therapy be effective?

The first of these questions was addressed by Deckers and colleagues (2001). In their study, patients with previously untreated generalised tonic–clonic and/or partial seizures were randomised to receive carbamazepine monotherapy (400 mg per day) or a combination of carbamazepine and valproate to give an equivalent drug load (200 and 300 mg per day, respectively). After one year of follow-up, no statistically significant differences were found between the two treatments in seizure frequency or side effects.

The second question was addressed in a pragmatic study in patients with partial epilepsy not controlled after single or sequential anti-epileptic monotherapies who were randomised to monotherapy with an alternative AED or to adjunctive therapy with a second AED (Beghi *et al.*, 2003). Overall there was no difference in efficacy or adverse events between those randomised to substitution versus those randomised to combination therapy. These studies thus provide no evidence for a benefit of combination therapy over monotherapy.

What if monotherapy has failed with two drugs, does a combination offer any advantage? This has been investigated in five studies (two exist only as proceedings reports) (Hakkarainen, 1980; Kanner and Frey, 2000; Rowan *et al.*, 1983; Tanganelli and Regesta, 1996; Walker and Koon, 1988). These studies suggest that patients respond to combinations of phenytoin and carbamazepine, carbamazepine and valproate, vigabatrin and carbamazepine, lamotrigine and valproate or valproate and ethosuximide when they have failed to respond to these drugs as monotherapies. These studies imply that people who have failed to respond to drugs as monotherapies may respond to combinations, interestingly this was seen not only for drugs that have different mechanisms of action, but also for drugs that have similar mechanisms of action (phenytoin and carbamazepine).

Are there specific drug combinations or add-on therapies that are more successful than others? Most of the data on this are uncontrolled, observational studies. Meta-analysis of randomised control trials suggest that there is no significant difference in efficacy between add-on medications in partial epilepsy, but overall levetiracetam seemed to have the best responder-withdrawal ratio (Marson *et al.*, 2001; Marson *et al.*, 1997).

This analysis is confounded by comparing across short-term trials that have different entry criteria and varying dosing regimens. What about studies of other forms of epilepsy? Lamotrigine, felbamate and topiramate have all demonstrated efficacy as add-on medication in Lennox-Gastaut syndrome (Hancock and Cross, 2003). There has been a paucity of randomised control trials in idiopathic generalised epilepsies (especially juvenile myoclonic epilepsy), probably because many patients become seizure free with monotherapy and these syndromes predominantly affect children.

Topiramate has been compared to placebo as add-on in juvenile myoclonic epilepsy, and was shown to significantly decrease secondary generalised seizures (the effects on other seizure types did not reach significance) (Biton and Bourgeois, 2005). A recently reported study of levetiracetam as add-on in drug-resistant idiopathic generalised epilepsy with myoclonic seizures (mostly juvenile myoclonic epilepsy) demonstrated impressive efficacy with 25% becoming free of myoclonic seizures (Verdu *et al.*, 2005). It is not certain whether this is due to the good efficacy of levetiracetam alone or in combination with other drugs since levetiracetam has been shown in a noninferiority trial to have similar efficacy to carbamazepine in monotherapy (Ben-Menachem *et al.,* 2006). This study lends support to similar findings in open-label studies (Grunewald, 2005).

Long-term retention studies in clinical practice may give a better idea of the success of a medication in combination. Such studies give a compound measure of the efficacy and adverse effects of a particular medication as add-on therapy. In studies from the same centre of retention rates of add-on medications at three years, levetiracetam was best (56% retention) followed by topiramate (30%, most withdrawals were due to adverse events), lamotrigine (29%) and gabapentin (<10%) (Depondt *et al.,* 2006; Lhatoo *et al.,* 2000). These studies did not highlight any particularly successful combinations, but another retention study confirmed that the combination of lamotrigine with valproate may be more successful than lamotrigine combined with other medication (Knoester *et al.,* 2005). In order to identify specific combinations, some have looked at the combinations that patients in a clinic are most likely to be taking. Such studies suffer in that the combinations that patients are taking may be influenced by the prejudices of the prescribing physician, but again these lend support to the efficacy of the combination of lamotrigine and valproate (Stephen and Brodie, 2002).

Although these studies support the use of certain combinations, we should be aware that combinations that are synergistic for efficacy may also be synergistic for adverse events. This is seen to some extent with lamotrigine and valproate in combination, which has a great propensity to cause tremor (Kanner and Frey, 2000) and which has a markedly increased teratogenic effect (Morrow *et al.,* 2006).

CONCLUSION

So what combinations are most likely to result in seizure freedom? The greatest evidence supports the use of lamotrigine and valproate; this combination demonstrates significant synergy in animal models, which is largely confirmed by human data. The drawback is that there may be increased side-effects. There are some data to support the contention that we should not be using a combination of two sodium channel antagonists. Beyond this there are no convincing data for specific combinations. We know that the new drugs are effective as add-on medications, and overall, at present, topiramate and levetiracetam seem in clinical practice to represent the most effective add-on medications in both partial and some generalised epilepsies.

REFERENCES

Beghi, E., Gatti, G., Tonini, C., Ben-Menachem, E., Chadwick, D. W., Nikanorova, M., Gromov, S. A., Smith, P. E., Specchio, L. M. and Perucca, E. (2003). Adjunctive therapy versus alternative monotherapy in patients with partial epilepsy failing on a single drug: a multicentre, randomised, pragmatic controlled trial. *Epilepsy Res* **57**, 1-13.

Ben-Menachem, E., Brodie, M. J. and Perucca, E. (2006). Efficacy of levetiracetam monotherapy; randomised, double-blind head to head comparison with carbamazepine-CR in newly diagnosed epilepsy patients with partial onset or generalised tonic-clonic seizures. *58th Annual Meeting of AAN;* San Diego, April 1-8. Abst. 509,006.

Biton, V. and Bourgeois, B. F. (2005). Topiramate in patients with juvenile myoclonic epilepsy. *Arch Neurol* **62**, 1705-1708.

Borden, L. A. (1996). GABA transporter heterogeneity: pharmacology and cellular localization. *Neurochem Int* **29**, 335-356.

Borowicz, K. K., Luszczki, J. J. and Czuczwar, S. J. (2004). Isobolographic and subthreshold analysis of interactions among felbamate and four conventional antiepileptic drugs in pentylenetetrazole-induced seizures in mice. *Epilepsia* **45**, 1176-1183.

Borowicz, K. K., Swiader, M., Luszczki, J. and Czuczwar, S. J. (2002). Effect of gabapentin on the anticonvulsant activity of antiepileptic drugs against electroconvulsions in mice: an isobolographic analysis. *Epilepsia* **43**, 956-963.

Bourgeois, B. F. (1986). Antiepileptic drug combinations and experimental background: the case of phenobarbital and phenytoin. *Naunyn Schmiedebergs Arch Pharmacol* **333**, 406-411.

Bourgeois, B. F. (1988a). Anticonvulsant potency and neurotoxicity of valproate alone and in combination with carbamazepine or phenobarbital. *Clin Neuropharmacol* **11**, 348-359.

Bourgeois, B. F. (1988b). Combination of valproate and ethosuximide: antiepileptic and neurotoxic interaction. *J Pharmacol Exp Ther* **247**, 1128-1132.

Bourgeois, B. F. and Wad, N. (1988). Combined administration of carbamazepine and phenobarbital: effect on anticonvulsant activity and neurotoxicity. *Epilepsia* **29**, 482-487.

Brodie, M. J. and Yuen, A. W. (1997). Lamotrigine substitution study: evidence for synergism with sodium valproate? 105 Study Group. *Epilepsy Res* **26**, 423-432.

Brooks-Kayal, A. R., Shumate, M. D., Jin, H., Rikhter, T. Y. and Coulter, D. A. (1998). Selective changes in single cell GABA(A) receptor subunit expression and function in temporal lobe epilepsy. *Nat Med* **4**, 1166-1172.

Buoni, S., Grosso, S. and Fois, A. (1999). Lamotrigine in typical absence epilepsy. *Brain Dev* **21**, 303-306.

Catterall, W. A. (1999). Molecular properties of brain sodium channels: an important target for anticonvulsant drugs. *Adv Neurol* **79**, 441-456.

Catterall, W. A. (2000a). From ionic currents to molecular mechanisms: the structure and function of voltage-gated sodium channels. *Neuron* **26**, 13-25.

Catterall, W. A. (2000b). Structure and regulation of voltage-gated Ca2+ channels. *Ann Rev Cell Dev Biol* **16**, 521-555.

Cipelletti, B., Avanzini, G., Vitellaro-Zuccarello, L., Franceschetti, S., Sancini, G., Lavazza, T., Acampora, D., Simeone, A., Spreafico, R. and Frassoni, C. (2002). Morphological organization of somatosensory cortex in Otx1(-/-) mice. *Neuroscience* **115**, 657-667.

Coulter, D. A., Huguenard, J. R. and Prince, D. A. (1989) Characterization of ethosuximide reduction of low-threshold calcium current in thalamic neurons. *Ann Neurol* **25**, 582-593.

Czuczwar, S. J. and Patsalos, P. N. (2001). The new generation of GABA enhancers. Potential in the treatment of epilepsy. *CNS Drugs* **15**, 339-350.

Davidson, D. T., Jr. and Berman, B. A. (1956). Phelantin for the treatment of epilepsy. *J Am Med Assoc* **160**, 766-768.

Deckers, C. L., Hekster, Y. A., Keyser, A., Meinardi, H. and Renier, W. O. (1997). Drug load in clinical trials: a neglected factor. *Clin Pharmacol Ther* **62**, 592-595.

Deckers, C. L., Hekster, Y. A., Keyser, A., Van Lier, H. J., Meinardi, H. and Renier, W. O. (2001). Monotherapy versus polytherapy for epilepsy: a multicenter double-blind randomized study. *Epilepsia* **42**, 1387-1394.

Depondt, C., Yuen, A. W., Bell, G. S., Mitchell, T., Koepp, M. J., Duncan, J. S. and Sander, J. W. (2006). The long term retention of levetiracetam in a large cohort of patients with epilepsy. *J Neurol Neurosurg Psychiatry* **77**, 101-103.

Grunewald, R. (2005). Levetiracetam in the treatment of idiopathic generalized epilepsies. *Epilepsia* **46 (Suppl 9)**, 154-160.

Hakkarainen, H. (1980). Carbamazepine vs. diphenylhydantoin vs. their combination in adult epilepsy. *Neurology* **30**, 354.

Hancock, E. and Cross, H. (2003). Treatment of Lennox-Gastaut syndrome. *Cochrane Database Syst Rev* CD003277.

Kanner, A. M. and Frey, M. (2000). Adding valproate to lamotrigine: a study of their pharmacokinetic interaction. *Neurology* **55**, 588-591.

Keros, S. and Hablitz, J. J. (2005). Subtype-specific GABA transporter antagonists synergistically modulate phasic and tonic GABAA conductances in rat neocortex. *J Neurophysiol* **94**, 2073-2085.

Klitgaard, H. (2001). Levetiracetam: the preclinical profile of a new class of antiepileptic drugs? *Epilepsia* **42 (Suppl 4)**, 13-18.

Knoester, P. D., Keyser, A., Renier, W. O., Egberts, A. C., Hekster, Y. A. and Deckers, C. L. (2005). Effectiveness of lamotrigine in clinical practice: results of a retrospective population-based study. *Epilepsy Res* **65**, 93-100.

Kohling, R., Konig, K., Lucke, A., Mayer, T., Wolf, P. and Speckmann, E. J. (2002). Prerather than co-application of vigabatrin increases the efficacy of tiagabine in hippocampal slices. *Epilepsia* **43**, 1455-1461.

Kuo, C. C. (1998). A common anticonvulsant binding site for phenytoin, carbamazepine, and lamotrigine in neuronal Na^+ channels. *Mol Pharmacol* **54**, 712-721.

Leresche, N., Parri, H. R., Erdemli, G., Guyon, A., Turner, J. P., Williams, S. R., Asprodini, E. and Crunelli, V. (1998). On the action of the anti-absence drug ethosuximide in the rat and cat thalamus. *J Neurosci* **18**, 4842-4853.

Lhatoo, S. D., Wong, I. C., Polizzi, G. and Sander, J. W. (2000). Long-term retention rates of lamotrigine, gabapentin, and topiramate in chronic epilepsy. *Epilepsia* **41**, 1592-1596.

Luszczki, J. J. and Czuczwar, S. J. (2003). Isobolographic and subthreshold methods in the detection of interactions between oxcarbazepine and conventional antiepileptics—a comparative study. *Epilepsy Res* **56**, 27-42.

Luszczki, J. J. and Czuczwar, S. J. (2004a). Isobolographic profile of interactions between tiagabine and gabapentin: a preclinical study. *Naunyn Schmiedebergs Arch Pharmacol* **369**, 434-446.

Luszczki, J. J. and Czuczwar, S. J. (2004b). Three-dimensional isobolographic analysis of interactions between lamotrigine and clonazepam in maximal electroshock-induced seizures in mice. *Naunyn Schmiedebergs Arch Pharmacol* **370**, 369-380.

Luszczki, J. J. and Czuczwar, S. J. (2005a). Interaction between lamotrigine and felbamate in the maximal electroshock-induced seizures in mice: an isobolographic analysis. *Eur Neuropsychopharmacol* **15**, 133-142.

Luszczki, J. J. and Czuczwar, S. J. (2005b). Isobolographic characterisation of interactions among selected newer antiepileptic drugs in the mouse pentylenetetrazole-induced seizure model. *Naunyn Schmiedebergs Arch Pharmacol* **372**, 41-54.

Luszczki, J., Swiader, M., Czuczwar, M., Kis, J. and Czuczwar, S. J. (2003a). Interactions of tiagabine with some antiepileptics in the maximal electroshock in mice. *Pharmacol Biochem Behav* **75**, 319-327.

Luszczki, J. J., Borowicz, K. K., Swiader, M. and Czuczwar, S. J. (2003b). Interactions between oxcarbazepine and conventional antiepileptic drugs in the maximal electroshock test in mice: an isobolographic analysis. *Epilepsia* **44**, 489-499.

Luszczki, J. J., Czuczwar, M., Kis, J., Krysa, J., Pasztelan, I., Swiader, M. and Czuczwar, S. J. (2003c). Interactions of lamotrigine with topiramate and first-generation antiepileptic drugs in the maximal electroshock test in mice: an isobolographic analysis. *Epilepsia* **44**, 1003-1013.

Luszczki, J. J., Swiader, M., Parada-Turska, J. and Czuczwar, S. J. (2003d). Tiagabine synergistically interacts with gabapentin in the electroconvulsive threshold test in mice. *Neuropsychopharmacology* **28**, 1817-1830.

Luszczki, J. J., Andres, M. M. and Czuczwar, S. J. (2005a). Synergistic interaction of gabapentin and oxcarbazepine in the mouse maximal electroshock seizure model—an isobolographic analysis. *Eur J Pharmacol* **515**, 54-61.

Luszczki, J. J., Wojcik-Cwikla, J., Andres, M. M. and Czuczwar, S. J. (2005b). Pharmacological and behavioral characteristics of interactions between vigabatrin and conventional antiepileptic drugs in pentylenetetrazole-induced seizures in mice: an isobolographic analysis. *Neuropsychopharmacology* **30**, 958-973.

Luszczki, J. J., Andres, M. M., Czuczwar, P., Cioczek-Czuczwar, A., Ratnaraj, N., Patsalos, P. N. and Czuczwar, S. J. (2006). Pharmacodynamic and pharmacokinetic characterization of interactions between levetiracetam and numerous antiepileptic drugs in the mouse maximal electroshock seizure model: an isobolographic analysis. *Epilepsia* **47**, 10-20.

Lynch, B. A., Lambeng, N., Nocka, K., Kensel-Hammes, P., Bajjalieh, S. M., Matagne, A. and Fuks, B. (2004). The synaptic vesicle protein SV2A is the binding site for the antiepileptic drug levetiracetam. *Proc Natl Acad Sci U S A* **101**, 9861-9866.

Maguire, J. L., Stell, B. M., Rafizadeh, M. and Mody, I. (2005). Ovarian cycle-linked changes in GABA(A) receptors mediating tonic inhibition alter seizure susceptibility and anxiety. *Nat Neurosci* **8**, 797-804.

Marson, A. G., Hutton, J. L., Leach, J. P., Castillo, S., Schmidt, D., White, S., Chaisewikul, R., Privitera, M. and Chadwick, D. W. (2001). Levetiracetam, oxcarbazepine, remacemide and zonisamide for drug resistant localization-related epilepsy: a systematic review. *Epilepsy Res* **46**, 259-270.

Marson, A. G., Kadir, Z. A., Hutton, J. L. and Chadwick, D. W. (1997). The new antiepileptic drugs: a systematic review of their efficacy and tolerability. *Epilepsia* **38**, 859-880.

Masuda, Y., Utsui, Y., Shiraishi, Y., Karasawa, T., Yoshida, K. and Shimizu, M. (1981). Evidence for a synergistic interaction between phenytoin and phenobarbital in experimental animals. *J Pharmacol Exp Ther* **217**, 805-811.

Mattson, R. H., Cramer, J. A., Collins, J. F., Smith, D. B., Delgado-Escueta, A. V., Browne, T. R., Williamson, P. D., Treiman, D. M., McNamara, J. O., McCutchen, C. B. *et al.* (1985). Comparison of carbamazepine, phenobarbital, phenytoin, and primidone in partial and secondarily generalized tonic-clonic seizures. *N Engl J Med* **313**, 145-151.

McCormick, D. A. and Contreras, D. (2001). On the cellular and network bases of epileptic seizures. *Annu Rev Physiol* **63**, 815-846.

Mclean, M. J. and Macdonald, R. L. (1986). Sodium valproate, but not ethosuximide, produces use- and voltage-dependent limitation of high frequency repetitive firing of action potentials of mouse central neurons in cell culture. *J Pharmacol Exp Ther* **237**, 1001-1011.

Mclean, M. J., Schmutz, M., Wamil, A. W., Olpe, H. R., Portet, C. and Feldmann, K. F. (1994). Oxcarbazepine: mechanisms of action. *Epilepsia* **35 (Suppl 3)**, S5-S9.

Mehta, A. K. and Ticku, M. K. (1999). An update on GABA$_A$ receptors. *Brain Res Rev* **29**, 196-217.

Morrow, J., Russell, A., Guthrie, E., Parsons, L., Robertson, I., Waddell, R., Irwin, B., Mcgivern, R. C., Morrison, P. J. and Craig, J. (2006). Malformation risks of antiepileptic drugs in pregnancy: a prospective study from the UK Epilepsy and Pregnancy Register. *J Neurol Neurosurg Psychiatry* **77**, 193-198.

Nusser, Z., Naylor, D. and Mody, I. (2001). Synapse-specific contribution of the variation of transmitter concentration to the decay of inhibitory postsynaptic currents. *Biophys J* **80**, 1251-1261.

Overstreet, L. S. and Westbrook, G. L. (2001). Paradoxical reduction of synaptic inhibition by vigabatrin. *J Neurophysiol* **86**, 596-603.

Overstreet, L. S. and Westbrook, G. L. (2003). Synapse density regulates independence at unitary inhibitory synapses. *J Neurosci* **23**, 2618-2626.

Pisani, F., Oteri, G., Russo, M. F., Di Perri, R., Perucca, E. and Richens, A. (1999). The efficacy of valproate-lamotrigine comedication in refractory complex partial seizures: evidence for a pharmacodynamic interaction. *Epilepsia* **40**, 1141-1146.

Poolos, N. P., Migliore, M. and Johnston, D. (2002). Pharmacological upregulation of h-channels reduces the excitability of pyramidal neuron dendrites. *Nat Neurosci* **5**, 767-774.

Remy, S. and Beck, H. (2006). Molecular and cellular mechanisms of pharmacoresistance in epilepsy. *Brain* **129**, 18-35.

Rowan, A. J., Meijer, J. W., De Beer-Pawlikowski, N., Van Der Geest, P. and Meinardi, H. (1983). Valproate-ethosuximide combination therapy for refractory absence seizures. *Arch Neurol* **40**, 797-802.

Rudolph, U. and Mohler, H. (2006). GABA-based therapeutic approaches: GABA$_A$ receptor subtype functions. *Curr Opin Pharmacol* **6**, 18-23.

Semyanov, A., Walker, M. C., Kullmann, D. M. and Silver, R. A. (2004). Tonically active GABA A receptors: modulating gain and maintaining the tone. *Trends Neurosci* **27**, 262-269.

Sills, G. J. (2006). The mechanisms of action of gabapentin and pregabalin. *Curr Opin Pharmacol* **6**, 108-113.

Sills, G. J., Butler, E., Thompson, G. G. and Brodie, M. J. (1999). Vigabatrin and tiagabine are pharmacologically different drugs. A pre-clinical study. *Seizure* **8**, 404-411.

Sills, G. J., Butler, E., Thompson, G. G. and Brodie, M. J. (2004). Pharmacodynamic interaction studies with topiramate in the pentylenetetrazol and maximal electroshock seizure models. *Seizure* **13**, 287-295.

Stephen, L. J. and Brodie, M. J. (2002). Seizure freedom with more than one antiepileptic drug. *Seizure* **11**, 349-351.

Tanganelli, P. and Regesta, G. (1996). Vigabatrin vs. carbamazepine monotherapy in newly diagnosed focal epilepsy: a randomized response conditional cross-over study. *Epilepsy Res* **25**, 257-262.

Van Rijn, C. M., Sun, M. S., Deckers, C. L., Edelbroek, P. M., Keyser, A., Renier, W. and

Meinardi, H. (2004). Effects of the combination of valproate and ethosuximide on spike wave discharges in WAG/Rij rats. *Epilepsy Res* **59**, 181-189.

Verdu, P., Wajgt, A., Schiemann Delgado, J. and Noachtar, S. (2005). Efficacy and safety of levetiracetam 3000 mg/d as adjunctive treatment in adolescents and adults suffering from idiopathic generalised epilepsy with myoclonic seizures. *Epilepsia* **46 (Suppl 6)**, S56-S57.

Walker, J. E. and Koon, R. (1988). Carbamazepine versus valproate versus combined therapy for refractory partial complex seizures with secondary generalization. *Epilepsia* **29**, 263.

White, H. S. (1999). Comparative anticonvulsant and mechanistic profile of the established and newer antiepileptic drugs. *Epilepsia* **40 (Suppl 5)**, S2-10.

Wu, Y., Wang, W. and Richerson, G. B. (2003). Vigabatrin induces tonic inhibition via GABA transporter reversal without increasing vesicular GABA release. *J Neurophysiol* **89**, 2021-2034.

Seizure Freedom: Clinical, Research and Quality of Life Perspectives
Edited by Michael R. Trimble
© 2006 Clarius Press Ltd

5

Seizure Freedom with Epilepsy Surgery

DAVID A. BELL and ANDREW M. McEVOY

*The National Hospital for Neurology and Neurosurgery
and Institute of Neurology,
Queen Square, London, UK*

INTRODUCTION

The discovery that surgery on the brain could render a patient seizure-free most likely dates back to 1886. Sir Victor Horsley's first epilepsy operation was performed on a Scotsman who had developed seizures following a depressed skull fracture (Paget, 1919). By the end of 1886 Horsley had performed 10 operations of which nine were judged successful (Horsley, 1886). Over the following 10 years approximately 400 epilepsy procedures were documented in the medical literature (Andriezen, 1894).

Wilder Penfield and his team performed the first temporal lobectomy for epilepsy in 1928 and in 1934 the Montreal Neurological Institute opened with the primary aim of advancing the understanding and management of epilepsy (Penfield and Flanigin, 1950). Penfield and Flanigin reported that of 68 temporal lobe resections performed between 1939 and 1949, seizure cure was obtained in over half of the patients. The past 50 years have seen dramatic advances in both the investigation and surgical treatment of seizures. In the 1980s the selective amygdalo-hippocampectomy was first described (Wieser and Yasargil, 1982) and the increasing benefit of disconnection procedures such as corpus callosotomy and hemispherectomy was recognised.

The 1990s have seen the emergence of vagus nerve stimulation (Penry and Dean, 1990) and multiple subpial transection (Morrell *et al.*, 1989) largely as palliative procedures. More recently gamma knife radiosurgery has been proposed as an alternative strategy to treat epilepsy of medial temporal origin (Regis, *et al.*, 1995; 1999; 2000).

The majority of patients with epilepsy will not undergo surgery. A cohort study in the United Kingdom demonstrated that over a 10-year period up to 3% of patients may be suitable candidates for surgery (Lhatoo *et al.*, 2003). All surgical procedures carry risks which need to be carefully considered and balanced against the potential benefits of either a reduction in seizure frequency or the chance of remission. In this chapter we will examine the surgical procedures currently available for the treatment of epilepsy. We shall specifically address the ability of different surgical interventions to render a patient seizure-free.

In order to do this we must consider what is meant by the term seizure-free? At what point in time can a patient be considered to be cured? Historical series have tended to report outcomes at one and two years, however it is has been recognised that there is a significant rate of relapse over longer periods of follow-up even in patients who appeared to be seizure-free. We shall therefore report on the long-term success rates both in terms of seizure freedom as well as seizure reduction. We shall also look at pre- and post-operative factors which may influence the long-term prognosis.

CLASSIFICATION OF THE RESULTS OF EPILEPSY SURGERY

Whilst it is recognised that outcome from surgery must incorporate complication rates as well as health related quality of life assessments, seizure freedom will be the most significant factor to be addressed. Although many different outcome classifications are in use, the most commonly used is that formulated at the Palm Desert Conference and listed below. This is commonly known as the Engel classification (Engel, 2005).

CLASS	DESCRIPTION
1	Free of disabling seizures
1A	Complete seizure freedom
1B	Non disabling simple partial seizures
1C	Some disabling seizures but seizure-free for two years
1D	Generalised convulsion on drug withdrawal only
2	Rare disabling seizures
2A	Initially free but now rare seizures
2B	Rare disabling seizures
2C	More than rare disabling seizures after surgery but rare seizures for at least two years
2D	Nocturnal seizures only
3	Worthwhile improvement
3A	Worthwhile seizure reduction
3B	Prolonged seizure-free intervals amounting to more than half the follow-up period but not less than two years
4	No worthwhile improvement
4A	Significant seizure reduction
4B	No appreciable change
4C	Seizures worse

Temporal Lobe Resection

Surgery on the temporal lobe may be subdivided into resections incorporating the hippocampus and amydala along with the temporal lobe (anterior temporal lobe resection), lesional surgery sparing the medial temporal structures (so called neocortical resection) and selective amygdalo-hippocampectomy.

The decision as to which procedure to use will depend on both the results of the preoperative work up and on the individual preference of the surgeon.

We shall discuss the results of these procedures individually.

Anterior temporal lobectomy

The most common seizure type occurring in adults is a complex partial seizure of mesial temporal lobe origin. The success rates of temporal lobe surgery for this condition have been extensively analysed particularly over the last 20 years. The majority of results published are based upon longitudinal series with varying lengths of follow up.

The first major series to look at quantitative outcomes following surgery was produced at the 1992 Palm Desert Conference (Engel, 2005). At this time 100 centres across the United States produced outcome results for 3,579 patients undergoing anterior temporal lobectomy (ATL) between 1986 and 1990. There were recognised difficulties in extrapolating results from multiple centres and therefore results were considered approximations. The reported rate of seizure freedom was 67.9% with a further 24.0% reporting an improvement in seizure frequency. The length of follow up and therefore durability of outcome over time was not reported.

Around this time a series of 100 patients undergoing ATL in a single unit was reported by Walczak and colleagues (2005). Mean follow up was nine years. Results were available for all patients at two years. They reported 63% of patients seizure-free. Interestingly 14 (22%) patients who were seizure-free at two years experienced seizures during the first post-operative year. The rationale for withdrawal of anti-epileptic drugs was not reported and it is not clear whether seizures in this group were generalised seizures secondary to withdrawal of medication. However, these data support previous evidence that, in a given patient, outcome cannot be established until at least one year post-operatively. The study noted that if seizure-free at one year, there was a 70% chance of being seizure-free at 10 years with this percentage rising to 80% if seizure-free at two years.

So and colleagues (1997) reported 184 patients undergoing ATL over a 3-year period in one centre. Follow-up was available for all patients at one year. Outcome was classified according to seizure frequency. Seizure freedom, either on or off medication, or non-disabling simple partial seizures were both classified as being a good outcome. At one year 78.3% of patients reported good outcome.

In 1999, Salanova reported a series of 145 patients treated over an 11-year period. 66% of patients were seizure-free at one year, 63% at two years. Twelve (55%) of 22 patients were seizure-free at 10-year follow-up (Salanova et al., 1999). Out of the 96 patients who were seizure-free at one year, 16 (17%) had recurrent seizures at the last follow-up. Only seven (8%) patients who were seizure-free at two years subsequently redeveloped seizures. Fifteen (31%) of the patients who continued to have seizures at one year subsequently became seizure-free for at least two years. This is recognised and referred to as a running-down phenomenon, first described by Rasmussen (Rasmussen and Branch, 1962). Previous work by the same group has identified that running down appears to correlate with the size of the epileptogenic focus (Salanova et al., 1996). Patients in the seizure-free group tended to have the smallest epileptogenic areas whereas those in the running down group had intermediate size epileptogenic areas which may extend into the lateral temporal and posterior temporal areas. This study then demonstrates well the durability of the results of ATL with the probability of continuing seizure-free, if seizure-free for one or two years, of 83% and 92% respectively.

Foldvary and colleagues (2000) published data on 79 consecutive patients undergoing ATL over a period of 22 years. All patients had at least two years follow-up. At one year 50 (63%) of the patients were seizure-free. 71% of these remained seizure-free at 10 years. 42 (53%) of the patients remained seizure-free at two years, of these, 84% remained seizure-free at 10 years. This study was limited by the lack of pathological analysis of resected hippocampi as well as a lack of detailed work up data regarding structural and functional neuroimaging along with video EEG.

The landmark study, certainly in terms of levels of evidence, was published by Wiebe and colleagues (2001). This was the first prospective, randomised controlled trial of surgery for temporal lobe epilepsy. Eighty patients with temporal lobe epilepsy whose seizures were poorly controlled with medication were randomly assigned to either surgery or continuing medical therapy for one year. To be eligible for the study patients had to have seizure semiology consistent with a focus within the temporal lobe and for seizures to have been present for at least one year. This had to be supported by EEG, MRI and neuropsychological assessments. At one year follow-up, 58% of surgical patients and 8% of medical patients were free of seizures impairing consciousness (p<0.001). The authors argue that, on the basis of their own work (Blume, 1994) and that of others (Salanova et al., 1999; So et al., 1997; Ficker et al., 1999), seizure outcome at one year is a durable predictor of long-term seizure freedom. The authors argue that surgery should be considered for patients with temporal lobe epilepsy of any cause. This statement has, however, been disputed due to the fact that 70% of patients in the surgical group had MRI evidence of mesial temporal sclerosis (Hoch and Cole, 2002). This subgroup of patients has been previously recognised as having a good outcome from resective surgery (Berkovic et al., 1995). The poor outcome in the medical arm of the trial has also been a matter of discussion.

In 2002, Kumlien and colleagues reported a retrospective series of 83 patients with temporal lobe epilepsy who were referred for evaluation in a comprehensive epilepsy centre (Kumlien et al., 2002). All patients had semiology consistent with a temporal lobe epileptogenic focus, along with concordant EEG recordings and MRI evidence of hippocampal sclerosis. Thirty six patients underwent temporal lobe resection, the remaining 47 were treated medically. Mean follow-up was 4.4 years in the surgical group compared with 3.4 years in the medical group. At last follow-up 26 (72%) patients in the surgical group were seizure-free compared to 11 (23%) of non-surgical patients (p<0.001).

Following this Salanova and colleagues published further work extending on their previously published series (Salanova et al., 2002). This series consisted of 215 consecutive patients undergoing surgery for temporal lobe epilepsy. This study compared patients who became seizure-free against those who did not, along with focusing on long-term mortality. Mean follow-up was seven years. Overall 89% of patients became either seizure-free or had rare seizures. The age of 29 years was used as an artificial cut-off to create older and younger sub-groups. No significant difference was found in terms of outcome with 69% of both groups being seizure-free a last follow-up. The duration of seizures prior to surgery was assessed and there was found to be a trend towards improved outcome if seizures has been present for less than 10 years; however, this was not statistically significant (p=0.08). No difference in outcome was found when left and right sided resections were compared. Overall three (2%) patients who became seizure-free died during the follow-up period, compared with eight (11.9%) who continued to have seizures (p<0.005). When the mortality for both of these groups was compared against standardised mortality rates (SMR) for the general population it was found that the seizure-free group did not differ significantly from the general population whereas in those who continued to suffer seizures, the SMR was significantly raised at 7.4 (95% CI 3.2-14.5). This study again demonstrated the efficacy of temporal lobe resection and confirmed the long-term benefits in terms of a reduction in mortality.

In 2003 the initial results of the Multicenter Study of Epilepsy Surgery were published (Spencer et al., 2003). This was a multicentre prospective study incorporating all patients over 12 years of age undergoing resective epilepsy surgery in terms of either temporal lobe resection or neocortical resection (as any neocortical resection including temporal neocortex). A total of 355 patients had at least one year of follow-up. 77% of patients undergoing temporal lobe resection achieved at least one year of seizure freedom during follow up compared with 56% of patients undergoing neocortical resection. Interestingly, however, more patients in the temporal lobe group suffered a relapse than those undergoing neocortical resection (24% versus 4%, p=0.02). All patients underwent quality of life, depression and anxiety assessments using the Quality Of Life In Epilepsy questionnaire (QOLIE) (Devinsky *et al.*, 1995). All scores rose substantially in the first three months following surgery even in patients suffering ongoing seizures. The score however remained constant in those who were seizure-free whereas in those who relapsed the score returned to baseline over the following 12-24 months. This study also demonstrates that resection including the medial temporal structures in appropriately selected patients, may produce better outcomes than neocortical temporal resection alone.

In 2004, McIntosh and colleagues published results on 325 patients undergoing temporal lobe resection in one unit (McIntosh *et al.*, 2004). Mean follow-up from surgery was 9.6+/– 4.2 years. Seizure freedom rates fell from 78.5% at three months to 67.4% at six months. At one year the probability of seizure freedom was 60.9%, falling to 47.7% at five years, 41% at 10 years and 36.8% at 15 years. In patients with histologically proven hippocampal sclerosis who were seizure-free at two years, 75.6% remained seizure-free at 10 years.

The same year, Paglioli and colleagues reported results on a series of 135 patients, all undergoing temporal lobe resection for hippocampal sclerosis (Paglioli *et al.*, 2004). Mean follow-up was 5.5 years. Operative technique was either anterior temporal lobectomy or selective amygdalo-hippocampectomy. Seizure freedom rates at one, two, five and 10 years were 85%, 77%, 74% and 66% respectively. No significant difference in outcome was found between patients undergoing the two different procedures. The higher rates of good outcome in this series are attributed to the highly selected population of clearly defined radiological hippocampal sclerosis along with concordant EEG, semiology and neuropsychology.

In 2005 the longer term results of the previously discussed Multicenter Study were published (Spencer *et al.*, 2005). This study again incorporated both medial and neocortical temporal resections. 339 patients had at least two years follow-up and of these 297 (87.6%) underwent mesial temporal lobe resections. 202 (68%) patients achieved at least a 2-year remission from seizures. The presence of hippocampal sclerosis on the MRI was significantly associated with remission. Of patients achieving remission, 25% subsequently relapsed over the next three years.

To summarise, temporal lobe resection, particularly mesial temporal lobe resection in carefully selected patients is a durable, validated procedure for the treatment of epilepsy of temporal lobe origin. Seizure freedom may be achieved in 50-60% of patients with a further 10-20% achieving a significant reduction in seizure frequency.

Neocortical temporal resections

A proportion of patients will be found to harbour discrete lesions within the temporal lobe whilst undergoing epilepsy investigations; these include neoplasms, which are typically low grade, cavernomas and cortical dysplasia. Assuming that semiology and EEG / telemetry are concordant then resection of the presumed epileptogenic focus may be performed without the loss of mesial temporal structures. This carries the presumed benefit of avoiding the risks to memory, mood and vision associated with more medial resections.

The results of focal neocortical resections have not been as extensively analysed as those of mesial resection.

In 2001 Schramm and colleagues published a series of 62 patients undergoing focal neocortical resections (Schramm *et al.*, 2001). Seizure outcome was classified using Engel's scale. Mean follow-up was 21.9 months, and two years of follow-up was available in 32 patients of whom 81% became seizure-free. In patients with neoplasms 89% achieved seizure freedom (Engel Class 1) at last follow up.

The Multicenter Study included 42 patients undergoing focal neocortical resections, and of these only 21 (50%) achieved a two year remission from seizures (Spencer *et al.*, 2005). The authors of this study noted that the worst outcome in their neocortical resection subgroup was not statistically different to those undergoing mesial resection, perhaps due to the small numbers undergoing neocortical surgery alone.

Selective amygdalo-hippocampectomy

The concept of selective resection of the amygdala and hippocampus, first described by Niemeyer in 1958 was popularised by Yasargil in the early 1980s (Wieser and Yasargil, 1982). Selective amygdalo-hippocampectomy aims to resect the mesial temporal structures whilst preserving functional neocortex. The theoretical benefit is that the limited neocortical resection reduces the post-operative neuropsychological deficit. This benefit has not been conclusively demonstrated in the literature, and the procedure is more technically challenging than the standard anterior temporal lobectomy.

Wieser and colleagues (2003) published the long term results of 361 patients who underwent selective amygdalo-hippocampectomy over a 24-year period. All patients underwent standard preoperative investigations and had been followed up for at least one year. In patients with histopathological evidence of hippocampal sclerosis, 79% were seizure-free at four years. This fell to 59% in patients without clear evidence of hippocampal sclerosis. In this series there were no deaths related to surgery. Complications occurred in 21 patients. These ranged from minor wound problems (0.44%) to major postoperative haemorrhage (1.1%) and hemiparesis (0.66%).

Complications of temporal lobe resection

Temporal lobe resection, the most commonly performed surgical procedure for the treatment of epilepsy, has been demonstrated to be a safe procedure in many studies. It is important however, that prior to any surgery, patients are informed of the specific risks of the procedure so that an informed decision can be made. Post-operative infection occurs in less than 5% of patients, with mortality from this procedure being well below 1%. The most common neurological deficit is an upper contralateral quandrantanopia which on formal visual field testing may be present in up to 10% of patients. Although this field loss is rarely recognised by patients, it may be severe enough in some patients to prevent them from obtaining a licence to drive (Manji and Plant, 2000). A contralateral hemiparesis or hemiplegia may occur in approximately 1% of cases, most commonly related to vascular injury rather than direct parenchymal damage.

It is well recognised that a proportion of patients will go on to develop depression, anxiety and, rarely, psychosis following temporal lobe surgery, but these are beyond the scope of this chapter.

Frontal lobe resection for epilepsy

Frontal lobe epilepsy is the second most common epilepsy syndrome that is referred for surgical management. These patients account for between five and 15% of those with symptomatic partial seizures (Williamson *et al.*, 1985; Laskowitz *et al.*, 1995). Frontal lobe seizures may have distinct semiology which facilitates localisation. Cases may be broadly divided into cases with a clear lesion and those with no demonstrable radiological abnormality. Lesional frontal lobe epilepsy accounts for approximately one third of all frontal lobe epilepsy.

Resection of focal frontal lesions may produce good results in selected patients. Zaatreh and colleagues reported results on 37 patients undergoing resective surgery for focal frontal tumours over a 14 year period (Zaatreh *et al.*, 2002). The most common tumour was oligodendroglioma. Average follow-up was 8.7 years. At last follow-up 13 (35.1%) patients were seizure-free or only had auras (Engel Class 1), with 12 (32.4%) patients with rare seizures (Engel Class 2). Patients with a good outcome (Engel Class 1 or 2) were compared with those having a poor outcome (Engel Class 3 or 4). Tumour histology, age at diagnosis and treatment were not found to be related to outcome.

Non-lesional frontal lobe resection may be performed in patients who have concordant semiology and EEG recordings. Results for frontal lobe resection in these circumstances vary, but appear to be poorer than for lesional frontal lobe surgery. It would appear that surgery for lesional frontal lobe epilepsy is associated with better outcome than non-lesional syndromes, but not as good as lesional temporal lobe surgery.

Favourable outcomes for frontal lobe epilepsy have varied widely in previous series from 23 to 80% (Laskowitz *et al.*, 1995; Swartz *et al.*, 1998; Fish *et al.*, 1993; Jobst *et al.*, 2000; Mosewich *et al.*, 2000; Ferrier *et al.*, 1999; Jansky *et al.*, 2000; Williamson *et al.*, 1985; Rasmussen, 1983; Shimizu, 1997; Salanova *et al.*, 1995). Larger studies in general report good outcomes in 50-55% of patients. The majority of these series were in non-lesional frontal lobe epilepsy.

Occipital lobe resection

Although rare in comparison to temporal and frontal lobe epilepsy, occipital epilepsy is well recognised as a distinct seizure type with typical semiology and characteristic imaging findings. Surgery for focal occipital lesions has been shown to produce good outcomes in carefully selected patients.

Occipital seizures can be difficult to localise with EEG and this may make decisions regarding surgery difficult, particularly in patients with normal MRI.

Kun and colleagues (2005) reported results on a series of 26 patients undergoing occipital lobe surgery over a seven year period. All patients underwent intracranial EEG monitoring to confirm seizure onset within the occipital lobe. Post-surgical follow up was greater than two years in all patients. Sixteen (61.5%) patients were seizure-free at two years. Visual field deficits were present in 21 patients post-operatively. Twenty patients in this series had evidence of cortical dysplasia on subsequent pathological analysis. Tumours were present in only two patients in this series.

Hemispheric disconnection – functional hemispherectomy

A small proportion of patients with chronic epilepsy will have diffuse disorders involving an extensive area of one hemisphere driving the epileptic focus. Disconnection of this hemisphere from the normal one may render the patient seizure-free. Total surgical resection of a hemisphere though technically possible, is associated with significant complications over time, the most recognised being superficial cerebral haemosiderosis (Oppenheimer and Griffith, 1966) and hydrocephalus. Thus in recent years this latter procedure has tended to be replaced by those which disconnect the hemisphere such as a functional hemispherectomy or hemispherotomy. These operations divide the major commissural fibres connecting the hemisphere to the deep grey matter structures and the contralateral hemisphere. The indications for this procedure include perinatal cerebral infarcts, Rasmussen's encephalitis and hemimegalencephaly. Disconnection of the hemisphere is associated with the development of predictable neurological outcome and is therefore most suitable for patients with pre-existing neurological deficits. In patients with only mild hemiparesis, surgery may be associated with a deterioration in limb function. This loss needs to be balanced against the benefits of surgery in terms of seizure control and social and intellectual development.

Patients undergoing dominant hemisphere disconnection before the age of five years may expect language function to be satisfactory but in older patients language function will be impaired by the procedure (Engel, 2005; Landau and Kleffner, 1957). However, in carefully selected patients seizure freedom in excess of 80% can be expected.

Palliative epilepsy surgery

A significant number of epilepsy patients will not be suitable candidates for resective surgery. This may be due to the fact that a seizure focus cannot be clearly localised, or due to a clear seizure focus being identified in an area which is not amenable to surgery. This is most commonly due to the fact that surgical resection will lead to unacceptable neurological deficit. In these circumstances procedures to try to disconnect the epileptogenic zone may be performed. These include multiple subpial transactions and corpus callosotomy. Vagus nerve stimulation uses electrical stimulation of the vagus nerve to modify seizure activity.

Multiple subpial transection (MST)

When the epileptogenic zone lies within an area of functionally critical cortex, resection may result in an unacceptable level of neurological deficit. The underlying principle of MST is that the functional arrangement of the cerebral cortex is primarily vertical whereas the intracortical fibres thought to be responsible for seizure spread are arranged horizontally. Morrell and colleagues (1989) devised the technique of passing a transector instrument at intervals of 4-5 mm perpendicular to the orientation of the gyrus. MST appears to have a specific role in this treatment of Landau-Kleffner syndrome. This condition of childhood is characterized by progressive loss of speech with a characteristic sleep EEG (Landau and Kleffner, 1957). MST has also been used in the primary motor cortex.

Spencer and colleagues (2002) published a series containing the results from four centres incorporating 211 operated cases. 75% of cases involved resection of focal cortical abnormalities as well as MST. This series reported 68% of patients undergoing lesion resection and MST as achieving a greater than 95% reduction in seizure frequency. This compared with 62% of patient undergoing MST alone.

Schramm and colleagues (2002) reported results on a series of 20 patients undergoing MST. Mean follow-up was 49 months with all patients being followed up for longer than one year. At last follow-up, one patient was seizure-free, one suffered less than two seizures per year and seven patients showed a greater than 75% reduction in seizure frequency. Several previous authors have reported much higher rates of seizure freedom; Liu (2000) reported seizure freedom in 63% of cases . All series looking at this procedure have been small and it would appear that the procedure carries a greater probability of reducing seizure frequency than achieving seizure freedom (Schramm *et al.*, 2002).

Corpus callosotomy

This procedure is generally reserved for the treatment of severe secondary generalised epilepsy which is characterised by frequent drop attacks which may cause injury and in whom medical therapy is ineffective. Patients may have other associated seizure types (Shorvon, 2005).

Short term seizure freedom may occur in up to 10% of patients but is rarely sustained. Satisfactory surgical outcome is usually defined as a greater than 50% reduction in seizure frequency. This is reported to occur in between 60-100% of series. Risks of the procedure include hemiparesis, incontinence and mutism which may be a consequence of frontal lobe retraction, and a disconnection syndrome which has often led the procedure to be performed in two stages. Overall the risks of severe permanent neurological damage are of the order of 5-10%. The efficacy and safety of vagus nerve stimulation in such patients has severely limited the indications for this procedure (Shorvon, 2005).

Vagus nerve stimulation

Vagus nerve stimulation (VNS) is a validated palliative procedure in the treatment of epilepsy particularly with idiopathic complex partial seizures. The procedure involves the insertion of stimulating electrodes around the left vagus nerve within the carotid sheath, coupled to a battery pack which is inserted into the subcutaneous space of the anterior chest wall. The stimulator frequency is tailored to the individual patient. The efficacy and safety of VNS has been established in a number of prospective randomised controlled trials (Ben Menachem *et al.*, 1994; DeGiorgio *et al.*, 2000; Handforth *et al.*, 1998; Ramsay *et al.*, 1994). These studies demonstrated an average seizure frequency reduction of 30% in patients receiving high stimulation compared with 11% in those receiving low stimulation (p=0.029) at 14 weeks follow-up. Seizure control appears to improve over time with a median seizure reduction of 45% at 12 months duration (DeGiorgio *et al.*, 2000). At this time 35% of patients had a greater than 50% reduction in seizure frequency with 20%

having a greater than 75% reduction in seizure frequency. Studies of longer duration have demonstrated a cumulative benefit with median seizure reductions of 52% at 12 year follow up (Uthman *et al.*, 2004).

Side effects of stimulation include hoarseness of the voice (56%), paraesthesiae (29%), dyspnoea (27%) and coughing (23%). No changes in gastric, pulmonary or cardiac function have been reported.

Stereotactic radiosurgery

Radiosurgery utilises multiple focused beams of radiation to produce destruction of small areas of cerebral tissue. It has been used most frequently in the treatment of arterio-venous malformations and in tumours. In vascular malformations radiosurgery has been demonstrated to produce seizure freedom in up to 90% of patients presenting with seizures as their primary complaint (Kida *et al.*, 2000).

Stereotactic radiosurgery has been proposed for the treatment of epilepsy caused by mesial temporal sclerosis. This was first performed by 1993 (Regis *et al.*, 1999) and is being evaluated in an ongoing study (Regis *et al.*, 2004). This study has demonstrated a rate of seizure freedom of 65% at two years, with similar complication rates to surgery in terms of mortality and morbidity.

CONCLUSION

This chapter has demonstrated that surgery, in carefully selected patients can produce excellent results in terms of seizure freedom or disease modification. The majority of patients with epilepsy will achieve seizure control with medication alone and will not be assessed for surgery. In patients with poorly controlled epilepsy the risks of surgery are acceptable particularly when compared to the risks of ongoing seizures and the potential side effects associated with long-term anticonvulsant usage.

REFERENCES

Andriezen, W.L. (1894). On some of the newer aspects of the pathology of insanity. *Brain* **18**, 548-692.

Ben Menachem, E., Manon-Espaillat, R., Ristanovic, R., Wilder, B.J., Stefan, H., Mirza, W. *et al.* (1994). Vagus nerve stimulation for treatment of partial seizures: 1. A controlled study of effect on seizures. First International Vagus Nerve Stimulation Study Group. *Epilepsia* **35**, 616-626.

Berkovic, S.F., McIntosh, A.M., Kalnins, R.M., Jackson, G.D., Fabinyi, G.C., Brazenor, G.A. *et al.* (1995). Preoperative MRI predicts outcome of temporal lobectomy: an actuarial analysis. *Neurology* **45**, 1358-1363.

Blume, W.T. (1994). Effectiveness of temporal lobectomy measured by yearly follow up and multivariate analysis. *J Epilepsy* **7**, 203-214.

DeGiorgio, C.M., Schachter, S.C., Handforth, A., Salinsky, M., Thompson, J., Uthman, B. *et al.* (2000). Prospective long-term study of vagus nerve stimulation for the treatment of refractory seizures. *Epilepsia* **41**, 1195-1200.

Devinsky, O., Vickrey, B.G., Cramer, J., Perrine, K., Hermann, B., Meador, K. *et al.* (1995). Development of the quality of life in epilepsy inventory. *Epilepsia* **36**, 1089-1104.

Engel, J.Jr. (2005) Surgical Treatment of the Epilepsies. Outcome with respect to epileptic seizures. 609-621.

Ferrier, C.H., Engelsman, J., Alarcon, G., Binnie, C.D., Polkey and C.E. (1999). Prognostic factors in presurgical assessment of frontal lobe epilepsy. *J Neurol Neurosurg Psychiatry* **66**, 350-356.

Ficker, D.M., So, E.L., Mosewich, R.K., Radhakrishnan, K., Cascino, G.D. and Sharbrough, F.W. (1999). Improvement and deterioration of seizure control during the postsurgical course of epilepsy surgery patients. *Epilepsia* **40**, 62-67.

Fish, D.R., Smith, S.J., Quesney, L.F., Andermann, F. and Rasmussen, T. (1993). Surgical treatment of children with medically intractable frontal or temporal lobe epilepsy: results and highlights of 40 years' experience. *Epilepsia* **34**, 244-247.

Foldvary, N., Nashold, B., Mascha, E., Thompson, E.A., Lee, N., McNamara, J.O. *et al.* (2000). Seizure outcome after temporal lobectomy for temporal lobe epilepsy: a Kaplan-Meier survival analysis. *Neurology* **54**, 630-634.

Handforth, A., DeGiorgio, C.M., Schachter, S.C. *et al.*, (1998). Vagus nerve stimulation therapy for partial-onset seizures: a randomized active-control trial. *Neurology* **51**, 48-55.

Hoch, D. and Cole, A.J. (2002). Surgery for Temporal-Lobe Epilepsy. *N Engl J Med* **346**, 292-295.

Horsley, V. (1886). Brain Surgery. *BMJ* 670-675.

Janszky, J., Jokeit, H., Schulz, R., Hoppe, M. and Ebner, A. (2000). EEG predicts surgical outcome in lesional frontal lobe epilepsy. *Neurology* **54**, 1470-1476.

Jobst, B.C., Siegel, A.M., Thadani, V.M., Roberts, D.W. and Rhodes, H.C. (2000). Williamson PD. Intractable seizures of frontal lobe origin: clinical characteristics, localizing signs, and results of surgery. *Epilepsia* **41**, 1139-1152.

Kida, Y., Kobayashi, T., Tanaka, T., Mori, Y., Hasegawa, T. and Kondoh, T. (2000). Seizure control after radiosurgery on cerebral arteriovenous malformations. *J Clin Neurosci* **7 (Suppl 1)**, S6-9.

Kumlien, E., Doss, R.C. and Gates, J.R. (2002). Treatment outcome in patients with mesial temporal sclerosis. *Seizure* **11**, 413-417.

Kun, L.S., Young, L.S., Kim, D.W., Soo, L.D. and Chung, C.K. (2005). Occipital lobe epilepsy: clinical characteristics, surgical outcome, and role of diagnostic modalities. *Epilepsia* **46**, 688-695.

Lhatoo, S.D., Solomon, J.K., McEvoy, A.W., Kitchen, N.D., Shorvon, S.D. and Sander, J.W. (2003). A prospective study of the requirement for and the provision of epilepsy surgery in the United Kingdom. *Epilepsia* **44**, 673-676.

Landau, W.M., Kleffner, F.R. (1957). Syndrome of acquired aphasia with convulsive disorder in children. *Neurology* **7**, 523-530.

Laskowitz, D.T., Sperling, M.R., French, J.A. and O'Connor, M.J. (1995). The syndrome of frontal lobe epilepsy: characteristics and surgical management. *Neurology* **45**, 780-787.

Liu Z. (2000). The surgical treatment of intractable epilepsy. *Stereotact Funct Neurosurg* **75**, 81-89.

McIntosh, A.M., Kalnins, R.M., Mitchell, L.A., Fabinyi, G.C., Briellmann, R.S. and Berkovic, S.F. (2004). Temporal lobectomy: long-term seizure outcome, late recurrence and risks for seizure recurrence. *Brain* **127**, 2018-2030.

Manji, H. and Plant, G.T. (2000). Epilepsy surgery, visual fields, and driving: a study of the visual field criteria for driving in patients after temporal lobe epilepsy surgery with a comparison of Goldmann and Esterman perimetry. *J Neurol Neurosurg Psychiatry* **68**, 80-82.

Morrell, F., Whisler, W.W. and Bleck, T.P. (1989). Multiple subpial transection: a new approach to the surgical treatment of focal epilepsy. *J Neurosurg* **70**, 231-239.

Mosewich, R.K., So, E.L., O'Brien, T.J., Cascino, G.D., Sharbrough, F.W., Marsh, W.R. *et al.* (2000). Factors predictive of the outcome of frontal lobe epilepsy surgery. *Epilepsia* **41**, 843-849.

Oppenheimer, D.R. and Griffith, H.B. (1966). Persistent intracranial bleeding as a complication of hemispherectomy. *J Neurol Neurosurg Psychiatry* **29**, 229-240.

Paget S. (1919) Sir Victor Horsley. Balliere, Tindall and Cox. London.

Paglioli, E., Palmini, A., Paglioli, E., da Costa, J.C., Portuguez, M., Martinez, J.V. *et al.* (2004). Survival analysis of the surgical outcome of temporal lobe epilepsy due to hippocampal sclerosis. *Epilepsia* **45**, 1383-1391.

Penfield, W. and Flanigin, H. (1950). Surgical therapy of temporal lobe seizures. *AMA Arch Neurol Psychiatry* **64**, 491-500.

Penry, J.K. and Dean, J.C. (1990). Prevention of intractable partial seizures by intermittent vagal stimulation in humans: preliminary results. *Epilepsia* **31 (Suppl 2)**, S40-S43.

Ramsay, R.E., Uthman, B.M., Augustinsson, L.E., Upton, A.R., Naritoku, D., Willis, J. *et al.* (1994). Vagus nerve stimulation for treatment of partial seizures: 2. Safety, side effects, and tolerability. First International Vagus Nerve Stimulation Study Group. *Epilepsia* **35**, 627-636.

Rasmussen, T. and Branch, C. (1962). Temporal lobe epilepsy; indications for and results of surgical therapy. *Postgrad Med* **31**, 9-14.

Rasmussen, T. (1983). Characteristics of a pure culture of frontal lobe epilepsy. *Epilepsia* **24**, 482-493.

Regis, J., Peragui, J.C., Rey, M., Samson, Y., Levrier, O., Porcheron, D. *et al.* (1995). First selective amygdalohippocampal radiosurgery for 'mesial temporal lobe epilepsy'. *Stereotact Funct Neurosurg* **64 (Suppl 1)**, S193-201.

Regis, J., Bartolomei, F., Rey, M., Genton, P., Dravet, C., Semah, F. *et al.* (1999). Gamma knife surgery for mesial temporal lobe epilepsy. *Epilepsia* **40**, 1551-1556.

Regis, J., Bartolomei, F., Rey, M., Hayashi, M., Chauvel, P. and Peragut, J.C. (2000). Gamma knife surgery for mesial temporal lobe epilepsy. *J Neurosurg* **93 (Suppl 3)**, S141-146.

Regis, J., Rey, M., Bartolomei, F., Vladyka, V., Liscak, R., Schrottner, O. *et al.* (2004). Gamma knife surgery in mesial temporal lobe epilepsy: a prospective multicenter study. *Epilepsia* **45**, 504-515.

Salanova, V., Morris, H.H., Van Ness, P., Kotagal, P., Wyllie, E. and Luders, H. (1995). Frontal lobe seizures: electroclinical syndromes. *Epilepsia* **36**, 16-24.

Salanova, V., Andermann, F., Rasmussen, T., Olivier, A. and Quesney, L. (1996). The running down phenomenon in temporal lobe epilepsy. *Brain* **119**, 989-996.

Salanova, V., Markand, O. and Worth, R. (1999). Longitudinal follow-up in 145 patients with medically refractory temporal lobe epilepsy treated surgically between 1984 and 1995. *Epilepsia* **40**, 1417-1423.

Salanova, V., Markand, O. and Worth, R. (2002). Temporal lobe epilepsy surgery: outcome, complications, and late mortality rate in 215 patients. *Epilepsia* **43**, 170-174.

Schramm, J., Kral, T., Grunwald, T. and Blumcke, I. (2001). Surgical treatment for neocortical temporal lobe epilepsy: clinical and surgical aspects and seizure outcome. *J Neurosurg* **94**, 33-42.

Schramm, J., Aliashkevich, A.F. and Grunwald, T. (2002). Multiple subpial transections: outcome and complications in 20 patients who did not undergo resection. *J Neurosurg* **97**, 39-47.

Shorvon S. (2004). The choice of drugs and approach to drug treatment in partial epilepsy. In: Shorvon, S.D., Perucca, E., Fish, D.E., Dodson, W.E. (Eds), *The Treatment of Epilepsy*. Blackwell Science (UK), 317-333.

So, E.L., Radhakrishnan, K., Silbert, P.L., Cascino, G.D., Sharbrough, F.W. and O'Brien, P.C. (1997). Assessing changes over time in temporal lobectomy: outcome by scoring seizure frequency. *Epilepsy Res* **27**, 119-125.

Spencer, S.S., Schramm, J., Wyler, A., O'Connor, M., Orbach, D., Krauss, G. *et al.* (2002). Multiple subpial transection for intractable partial epilepsy: an international meta-analysis. *Epilepsia* **43**, 141-145.

Spencer, S.S., Berg, A.T., Vickrey, B.G., Sperling, M.R., Bazil, C.W., Shinnar, S. *et al.* (2003). Initial outcomes in the Multicenter Study of Epilepsy Surgery. *Neurology* **61**, 1680-1685.

Spencer, S.S., Berg, A.T., Vickrey, B.G., Sperling, M.R., Bazil, C.W., Shinnar, S. *et al.* (2005). Predicting long-term seizure outcome after resective epilepsy surgery: the multicenter study. *Neurology* **65**, 912-918

Swartz, B.E., Delgado-Escueta, A.V., Walsh, G.O., Rich, J.R., Dwan, P.S., DeSalles, A.A. *et al.* (1998). Surgical outcomes in pure frontal lobe epilepsy and foci that mimic them. *Epilepsy Res* **29**, 97-108.

Uthman, B.M., Reichl, A.M., Dean, J.C., Eisenschenk, S., Gilmore, R., Reid, S. *et al.* (2004). Effectiveness of vagus nerve stimulation in epilepsy patients: a 12-year observation. *Neurology* **63**, 1124-1126.

Walczak, T.S. (2005). Anterior Temporal Lobectomy for Complex Partial Seizures: Evaluation,results and long term follow up in 100 cases. *Neurology* **40**, 413-418.

Wiebe, S., Blume, W.T., Girvin, J.P. and Eliasziw, M. (2001). A randomized, controlled trial of surgery for temporal-lobe epilepsy. *N Engl J Med* **345**, 311-318.

Wieser, H.G. and Yasargil, M.G. (1982). Selective amygdalohippocampectomy as a surgical treatment of mesiobasal limbic epilepsy. *Surg Neurol* **17**, 445-457.

Wieser, H.G., Ortega, M., Friedman, A. and Yonekawa, Y. (2003). Long-term seizure outcomes following amygdalohippocampectomy. *J Neurosurg* **98**, 751-763.

Williamson, P.D., Spencer, D.D., Spencer, S.S., Novelly, R.A. and Mattson, R.H. (1985). Complex partial seizures of frontal lobe origin. *Ann Neurol* **18**, 497-504.

Winston, K.R., Welch, K., Adler, J.R. and Erba, G. (1992). Cerebral hemicorticectomy for epilepsy. *J Neurosurg* **77**, 889-895.

Zaatreh, M.M., Spencer, D.D., Thompson, J.L., Blumenfeld, H., Novotny, E.J., Mattson, R.H. *et al.* (2002). Frontal lobe tumoral epilepsy: clinical, neurophysiologic features and predictors of surgical outcome. *Epilepsia* **43**, 727-733.

Seizure Freedom: Clinical, Research and Quality of Life Perspectives
Edited by Michael R. Trimble
© 2006 Clarius Press Ltd

6

Seizure Freedom
in Children

RICHARD APPLETON

Royal Liverpool Children's NHS Trust,
Alder Hey, Eaton Road,
Liverpool, UK

INTRODUCTION

Epilepsy is the most common and also the most chronic neurological disorder encountered in both children and adults. The drug and non-drug treatment of paediatric and adult epilepsy is very similar and it would seem reasonable to assume – and argue – that, whatever the age, seizure freedom without adverse side-effects from treatment, would be a common objective for the patient, their family and also the clinical team looking after them. However, despite these similarities, it is worth emphasising the significant differences that exist between epilepsy arising in childhood and that arising in adult life – if only because a number of these differences may influence the overall approach to the management of epilepsy and specifically the approach to, and likelihood of, achieving seizure freedom in children as compared to adults. These differences include (in children):

- heterogeneous group of conditions:
    many epilepsy syndromes
    many causes
    many prognoses
- generically (when naively considering epilepsy as a single 'condition'), most cases are idiopathic;
- frequently associated with additional problems (physical or learning difficulties, or both);

- not a static condition (evolves and changes with age; early age of onset typically associated with frequent and drug-resistant seizures in the first decade of life);
- not necessarily a life-long condition;
- treatment must take account of educational issues and family dynamics;
- unclear and inconsistent relationship between seizures and learning/behavioural difficulties;
- consideration of the effects of anti-epileptic drugs (AEDs) on the immature, developing brain.

It is the identification of the specific epilepsy syndrome, or where this is not possible, the seizure type (or types), that provides useful information on the probability of finding an underlying cause but more importantly, the prognosis of the epilepsy – and specifically:

- the likelihood of achieving seizure freedom (with AEDs) – the child will stop having seizures;
- the likelihood of the epilepsy entering a spontaneous remission – and the child being 'cured' of the epilepsy.

SEIZURE FREEDOM

What is seizure freedom?

An important question and one that is difficult to answer, and also define. Scientific studies often define seizure freedom as six, 12 or 24 months of having no seizures when reporting either spontaneous remission of seizures (i.e.: the natural history of the epilepsy) or when evaluating the response to one or more antiepileptic drugs in randomised controlled trials (RCTs). This is a relatively crude definition – as well as being generic – as it takes no account of the specific epilepsy syndrome, and, in those syndromes characterised by multiple seizure types (e.g. Lennox-Gastaut syndrome, severe myoclonic epilepsy in infancy), seizure freedom should ideally be addressed for each individual seizure type. This may be quite important for the child, as well as the family and the clinician, as being free of the major (tonic-clonic, atonic and tonic) seizures may be an 'acceptable' objective, even though other, more minor (absence, focal, brief myoclonic) seizures may persist.

Over the last 10-15 years, considerable attention has focused on the phenomenon of 'quality of life' in patients with epilepsy, with the design and publication of numerous (and still increasing) scales and measures (Baker *et al.*, 1998; Chapter 12 - this book). Predictably, seizure frequency (and therefore, seizure freedom) as well as seizure type tend to be constant domains or factors within these measures; however, there have been many other factors that have been included to try and assess a patient's, and in children their family's, quality of life. Not surprisingly, seizure type and seizure frequency remain the two most important factors that are closely correlated with, and appear to largely determine, a person's quality of life, whether these assessments are general or epilepsy-specific.

Finally, for most children and their families, a working definition of seizure freedom would probably be having no seizures (of any type) for as long as possible so that it allows them to live as full and unrestricted lives as possible.

Can seizure freedom be predicted?

There is considerable literature on seizure outcome and specifically seizure freedom, in children with epilepsy, but unfortunately much of these data are derived from selected groups (often from tertiary centres) that do not necessarily reflect or represent the situation in the general paediatric epilepsy population. The National Dutch Study of Epilepsy in Childhood is an impressive project that, through excellent collaboration between the paediatric neurologists in the Netherlands, has been able to provide population-based and long-term, detailed data on a cohort of all newly-diagnosed children with epilepsy, with a reported ascertainment of at least 96%. In this national cohort of newly-diagnosed children, 76% and 64% of 453 children had been seizure-free for 12 and 24 months respectively after five years of follow up (Arts *et al.*, 2004). The study also provided more detailed data of 12-month remission rates after two and five years of follow-up for the different epilepsy syndromes. It will be extremely useful to continue monitoring this cohort of children as they mature through adolescence and into adult life.

In children, unlike in adults, there is an extremely wide range of seizure control (in this situation defined as seizure freedom for a minimum of 12 months), depending on the specific epilepsy syndrome:

- migrating partial seizures of infancy: chance of seizure freedom: <5%
- West syndrome (irrespective of cause): chance of seizure freedom: 60+%
- Lennox-Gastaut syndrome: chance of seizure freedom: <5%
- severe myoclonic epilepsy in infancy chance of seizure freedom: 5-10%
- childhood-onset absence epilepsy: chance of seizure freedom: 65-70%
- benign partial epilepsy with centro-temporal spikes: chance of seizure freedom: 90+%
- juvenile myoclonic epilepsy
  treated with medication: chance of seizure freedom: 85+%
  untreated: chance of seizure freedom: 40%

- cryptogenic partial: chance of seizure freedom: 70%
- symptomatic partial: chance of seizure freedom: <50%
- unclassifiable: chance of seizure freedom: 50%

These data are based on the data published by Arts and colleagues (Arts *et al.*, 2004) and the author's experience in a tertiary epilepsy centre.

Although it is usually the specific epilepsy syndrome (or in the absence of a clearly-identified syndrome, the seizure type or types) and the underlying cause that primarily predict the likelihood of achieving seizure freedom, there may be other, contributory – and conflicting – factors. One example is child-hood-onset absence epilepsy where, despite meeting the ILAE-agreed electroclinical criteria and receiving optimal anti-epileptic medication, at least 30% of children will never achieve seizure freedom, or enter a sponta-neous remission. In part this could be explained by a mis-classification of the absences as generalised when in fact they may be focal, arising from the frontal lobes. However, genetic factors are likely to contribute to this poor response and the development of what is then regarded as a 'refractory epilepsy'. This pharmaco-resistance in epilepsy, and the wider phenomenon of 'pharmaco-genetics', is being studied extensively and a number of genetic polymorphisms have already been identified as being responsible for drug resistance. The pathophysiology of drug resistance is unclear but the current hypotheses include both an over-expression of multi-drug transporter proteins and alteration of target-sensitivity (the epileptogenic brain) to the antiepileptic drug(s) (Schmidt and Löscher, 2005; see also Chapter 8 – this book). Finally, it is unlikely that even if clear associations are identified between one or more polymorphisms and poor seizure control this would be of any day-to-day practical value. This is because, by necessity, all newly-presenting children with a specific epilepsy syndrome would have to be screened for these polymorphisms to try and identify those children who are unlikely to respond to a specific drug – and this has clear ethical and practical implications.

Who wants the child to be seizure-free?

An important question and one that is commonly overlooked, because the patient who is seizing is a child who is either unable to give an opinion, or is not always asked for their opinion – by anyone, including their doctor(s). The different people who may have 'something to say' and, consequently, may have an impact in this situation are many:

- the child;
- their parents;
- their grandparents;

- their siblings;
- the schoolteachers;
- the school nurse;
- the general practitioner;
- the paediatrician/paediatric neurologist;
- the nurse specialist in epilepsy;
- the psychologist.

Opinions expressed by these people are not always appropriate or justified and, as would be expected, each of the above may approach epilepsy and its management from different directions and with different agendas. Predictably, there are likely to be realistic but also unrealistic expectations, firstly about the effect of persisting seizures on the child's health, cognition/behaviour and leisure activities and secondly, on seizure control, including achieving seizure freedom.

Parents will generally find it very uncomfortable or distressing (and occasionally even shocking) to be told that their child has epilepsy; this may also be true of the children themselves, although usually to a far lesser extent. The family's initial response to the diagnosis will, at least in part, reflect what they already know or have seen (including on television) or heard about 'epilepsy', whether they have friends or family with the condition, and their own personality. Whatever their background and understanding there are likely to be a number of common – and entirely understandable – questions or themes:

- can he die from it?
- will the seizures cause brain damage?
- what causes it?
- will he be able to live a 'normal' life?
- will he able to go to (a 'normal') school?
- what will happen in the (his) future?
- can the seizures be stopped?
- will the 'epilepsy' ever go away?

These questions and issues emphasise the importance of not only adopting a comprehensive approach to the diagnosis of epilepsy as outlined above (and described in detail in the proposed revised classification of the International League Against Epilepsy [ILAE]) (Engel, 2001) but also ensuring that the diagnosis and management of epilepsy in children be supervised by paediatricians, paediatric neurologists and nurse specialists/practitioners who are trained, experienced and interested in epilepsy (National Institute for Health and Clinical Excellence, 2004; Scottish Intercollegiate Guidelines Network, 2005).

It is stating the obvious that the management of children must be holistic and must consider not just the seizures, but the child; how they function at home and in school; their role within the family and their peer group and their own feelings and perceptions about 'their' epilepsy. It is also clear that for many children, social and psychological factors outweigh the problem of preventing the seizures, even when the seizures are relatively easy to control. It is also very important to appreciate that for many parents, seizure control (and in reality this implies seizure freedom) is the over-riding objective and comes to dominate not only their own life, but also that of their child and siblings. As a consequence this may lead to inappropriate and constrictive parenting and even overt pathological sickness behaviour. In this situation the clinician has a crucial role in:

- ensuring that correct diagnoses of the epilepsy syndrome and underlying cause have been identified – and, consequently,
- providing accurate advice about the future prognosis – and,
- giving honest and realistic – and not inappropriately optimistic or pessimistic – information about achieving seizure freedom as soon as this is possible;
- explaining that even if a specific epilepsy syndrome is identified (and where the seizures are usually controlled in this syndrome), there is no guarantee that anti-epileptic medication will completely control the seizures;
- discussing the fact that, in most epilepsy syndromes in childhood, the use of anti-epileptic drugs will not affect the natural history of their child's epilepsy and influence whether or not their seizures will eventually remit;
- understanding and identifying those rare epilepsy syndromes, often called the 'epileptic encephalopathies', where there appears to be a relatively close correlation between seizure control (and improvement of the EEG) and developmental and cognitive outcome (e.g. West syndrome, severe myoclonic epilepsy in infancy, Landau-Kleffner syndrome and electrical status epilepticus of slow sleep [ESESS], Rasmussen syndrome). In these electro-clinical syndromes, management tends to be more aggressive in optimising the child's cognitive potential;
- considering the possibility that a surgical option may be possible and referring sooner rather than later. Excluding vagus nerve stimulation (VNS) and 'disconnection' procedures, a surgical resection of epileptogenic tissue offers the only therapeutic option that could potentially cure a child's epilepsy – although this can also never be guaranteed (Schmidt et al. 2004);

- emphasising that trying to control their child's seizures should not be the only objective and certainly not at the expense of the child's ability to function, grow and develop and enjoy life.

Unfortunately this ideal objective is often far easier said than done. In addition, when discussing epilepsy and its management with the family, citing evidence from studies, including from 'scientific', randomised controlled or good epidemiological studies, may be considered as irrelevant for an individual family, as they want to know what will happen to just one child – their own, unique child.

For the child who never achieves seizure freedom, despite optimal management and early, accurate and realistic counselling that seizure freedom is unlikely, a minority of parents will continue to pursue this objective; this is sometimes termed the 'Holy Grail' phenomenon. This may involve not only requesting that their child receive all available antiepileptic drugs (including those only available outside the UK), but demanding other medical opinions both within the UK, but also abroad (typically the USA). Parents will frequently ask if there is "an operation that can cure our child's epilepsy", and where this is not feasible will then frequently try complementary and alternative medicines (CAMs). The most common of these tend to include homeopathy, cranial osteopathy, non-ketogenic diets and faith-healing. As stated previously, the paediatrician's and paediatric neurologist's primary responsibility is to the child and any CAMs that may be detrimental to the child or significantly interfere with conventional treatment should be discouraged – and with a clear explanation about why these complementary therapies might be harmful to their child.

Finally, the doctor's (the general practitioner's or the hospital specialist's, or both) perception of, and approach to, seizure freedom is also likely to be important and consequently this may bias the family's own perceptions and expectations. It may be very frustrating for the doctors if their patient's seizures are not fully controlled, and this, together with the family's own response to their child's ongoing seizures may understandably put them under significant pressure – which may then influence management decisions. In this situation, it is relatively easy to focus exclusively on the child's seizures, and 'lose sight of the child' - to their detriment. One could justifiably argue that this runs the risk of treating not the child, but their parents and even the doctor(s).

WHAT IS THE EFFECT OF PERSISTENT SEIZURES?

Persisting seizures and the lack of seizure freedom may have significant – including major – medical, cognitive, psychological and economic effects on both the child and their family, even when the child's carers have 'accepted' their child's condition and have been able to adopt a positive and adjusted approach to a chronic illness and its consequences.

There is no doubt that persisting seizures and particularly, but not exclusively tonic-clonic seizures, typically, but not exclusively in children with moderate or severe learning difficulties, increases the risk of physical injury (accidents, burns, drowning) (Kemp and Sibert, 1993; Kirsch and Wirrell, 2001; Wirrell *et al.*, 1996; Ziegler *et al.*, 1994) and premature death, including sudden unexplained death in epilepsy (SUDEP); fortunately, these risks appear to be considerably lower than those seen in adults and are far more commonly seen in children with a symptomatic epilepsy, and usually when the child has additional physical or educational, difficulties, or both (Callenbach *et al.*, 2001; Camfield *et al.*, 2002; Appleton, 2003; see also Chapter 7 – this book).

There is evidence (occasionally controversial), that persisting seizures may adversely affect cognitive function and educational attainments, and, consequently career and employment potential and opportunities (Bourgeois, 1998; see also Chapter 10 – this book). Persisting and frequent abnormal electrical activity (particularly spike and wave but also sharp wave activity) in the absence of any obvious clinical seizure activity (sensory, motor or autonomic features) may also contribute to cognitive stagnation and even regression. This is more likely in the epileptic encephalopathies, and specifically, in West syndrome (demonstrating hypsarrhythmia, a form of electrical or non-convulsive status epilepticus on EEG); in continuous slow, spike and slow wave activity in the rare Landau-Kleffner syndrome and with electrical status epilepticus of slow wave sleep [ESESS]) (Dulac, 2001). There is also evidence that early-onset seizures occurring in the immature brain, even when this is not one of the recognised 'epileptic encephalopathies' described above, may have adverse effects on brain development, and consequently, brain function – although the precise pathophysiology of such effects remain unclear (Holmes *et al.*, 1999). Finally, persistent spike and wave or spike/sharp activity on EEG without any obvious clinical seizure activity but with cognitive dysfunction (concentration and memory problems), sometimes called 'transient cognitive impairment' (TCI) or, far less appropriately, 'sub-clinical seizure activity' is an important but controversial subject that falls outside the remit of this chapter on 'seizure freedom', which by current understanding must include some clinical manifestation.

In most situations, persisting seizures (as occurs in chronic, uncontrolled epilepsy) are likely to have significant detrimental social and psychological effects on both the child and the family. The unpredictability of attacks characteristically leads parents to describe the situation as like a 'time bomb just waiting to go off' or 'having to put their life on hold' and not allowing themselves to hope that the epilepsy might actually, eventually, be controlled and even enter a permanent remission. The psychological effects of such uncertainty and fear are obvious and it is not surprising that many families feel unable to get on with both their own life, as well as those of their other children. Studies have predictably confirmed what is well-recognised in clinical practice – that persisting seizures in a child are typically associated with high levels of anxiety and, consequently, with a reduced quality of life (Williams *et al.*, 2003). Families commonly become isolated, distancing themselves from their extended family, friends and the community. This is clearly a very difficult, if not potentially pathological situation and demands not only a holistic approach to management, but an approach that puts their child's seizures into perspective. Parents' networks and voluntary organisations may be very helpful, but only through help and support that is tailored for (and therefore accepted by), the individual family. How the family, but also the community (including the child's school and the child's friends) respond to the lack of seizure freedom will largely determine the severity of these effects.

In the young person, persistent seizures, even occurring on an infrequent basis may have a significant detrimental effect on their lifestyle, ambitions and consequently, their 'quality of life'. This will include precluding their ability to drive (unless their seizures have only occurred during sleep for a minimum of three years), and certain career choices, and not only those with relatively strict entry criteria (the armed services, police, fire and ambulance services, airline pilots, heavy goods vehicle and train drivers) – but also many others, depending upon the degree of seizure control, and the type(s) of seizures.

The opportunity of obtaining a driving licence frequently provides the teenager and young person with the most effective motivation for consistent adherence to taking their antiepileptic medication in the hope of becoming, and remaining, seizure-free. Limited evidence also suggests that, perhaps not unexpectedly, epilepsy having an onset in childhood and persisting into adult life, even if seizures are well controlled (including being seizure-free for five years) on antiepileptic medication may have significant detrimental effects; these include lower scores on general but also epilepsy-specific quality of life measures, higher rates of unemployment and lower socioeconomic status (Sillanpää *et al.*, 2004; see also Chapter 12 – this book).

Finally, any detrimental social and psychological effects on a family's functioning, as well as the effect of ongoing seizures and how it affects the child's health, are likely to adversely affect the family's ability to work – whether remaining in, or finding new employment or even if considering further education. Consequently, this may have an impact on the economic health of not just the individual family, but of the entire community.

WHAT IS THE EFFECT OF OVER-TREATMENT OF SEIZURES?

Inevitably, in attempting to control a child's seizures and render him seizure-free, there will be the risk of over-treatment, both in terms of the individual dosage(s) of the anti-epileptic drugs and the number of drugs that may be prescribed simultaneously and the almost exclusive focus of management on the seizures, rather than the child and his ability to function (Holmes, 2002).

Increasing the dose of an AED: Many of the AEDs have a recognised dose-range, including the recommended maximum dose. In children under 12 years of age dosing is usually based on body weight; adult doses tend to be based on the total daily dose. When an initial AED appears to be improving seizure control, it is generally reasonable to increase the dose of the drug until either seizure control (i.e. seizure freedom) is achieved or unacceptable side-effects develop. This occasionally necessitates a therapeutic compromise – achieving as good seizure control as possible (and particularly of any major or injury-inducing seizures) without any unacceptable side-effects. Unfortunately, this compromise is often difficult to achieve in practice. There is always the temptation to increase the dose 'just a little bit more', in an attempt to reach that all-elusive goal of seizure freedom. In so doing, some side-effects, typically on concentration, short-term memory and other cognitive impairments may develop quite subtly and therefore not be recognised. The encephalopathy associated with sodium valproate (VPA) may present acutely but may also present more insidiously, and its manifestations may be initially ascribed to either the child's frequent seizures or the persistently abnormal EEG or the possibility of an underlying degenerative disorder. Conversely, encephalopathic-like symptoms (ataxia, blurred vision, poor concentration) may be falsely ascribed to the effects of an AED when the child may have an underlying and progressive disorder (e.g. late infantile neuronal ceroid lipofuscinosis, Unverricht-Lundborg disease or Lafora body disease); in this situation it is important to recognise the specific side-effects of the individual antiepileptic drugs and correctly differentiate them from an alternative cause.

In the author's experience, increases in the dose of some anti-epileptic drugs, may paradoxically increase seizure frequency, which, for the inexperienced clinician may lead to further dose increases, with inevitable consequences. Finally, it is worth emphasising that, in adults (and there should be no reason to expect the same in children), there is little evidence that dose increments in patients receiving doses within the average to high/average range, results in seizure freedom in a large proportion of cases (Kwan and Brodie, 2001).

Adding a second anti-epileptic drug: It is always far easier to add another AED than to withdraw one and even if the addition of a new AED has rendered the child seizure-free, there is often a general reluctance to then withdraw the ineffective drug. Although it is recognised that a number of children with a range of epilepsy syndromes may require two maintenance AEDs to achieve acceptable seizure control, including seizure freedom, there is no evidence that in children, three (or more) drugs used simultaneously will significantly improve seizure control. In addition there are certain drugs or combinations of drugs that may be inappropriate for certain seizure types and may consequently exacerbate seizure control. This may lead to a diagnosis of 'intractable' epilepsy – with all the associated consequences outlined above. However, once the appropriate medication has been prescribed, the child may then become seizure-free.

Specific examples include;

- mis-diagnosing the prolonged absences (during which the child may be able to continue performing certain, even relatively complicated activities) of juvenile-onset absence epilepsy with complex partial seizures; the use of carbamazepine or oxcarbazepine in these children typically exacerbates the seizures, including provoking absence status. If this situation is not recognised, an additional drug might then be prescribed in the belief that two AEDs may be more effective – which may further exacerbate the problem and a spiralling deterioration in both seizure frequency but also the child's cognitive and behavioural functioning;

- not asking the teenager who has presented with her first tonic-clonic seizure after a late night party about whether she has early morning 'jerks' (myoclonic seizures), often noticed by the family and ignored by the teenager or absences, often noticed by her friends; again, the use of carbamazepine or oxcarbazepine (that will probably control the tonic-clonic seizures) may also result in myoclonic or absence status in this young person.

Other drugs may also result in deteriorating seizure control, even when this would not be anticipated from the drug's presumed mechanism of action, reported spectrum of activity and pharmacodynamic profile. One large retrospective study of over one thousand patients with focal (partial) epilepsy found that topiramate and vigabatrin were the drugs most commonly associated with a worsening of seizures, despite the fact that they are generally considered to be very effective in treating focal seizures (Elger et al.,1998).

These issues again emphasise the importance of ensuring that children with epilepsy are managed by knowledgeable and experienced clinicians to minimise these problems.

FAMILY PERSPECTIVES

It is relatively easy to write on seizure freedom from a somewhat 'cold' and understandably detached medical view point; the view or perspective from a family who have a child with epilepsy, particularly an epilepsy that is characterized by seizures that are hard to control, could be so much more illuminating and informative......

"Every caring parent wants their offspring to have a happy, healthy and content journey through childhood, adolescence and into adulthood, with the opportunity to reach their potential overcoming obstacles through knowledge acquisition and growing independence. For the parents of a child with a disabling or chronic medical condition, the desires are just the same but the obstacles are more difficult to overcome.

"As parents of a daughter with a form of epilepsy that is not completely controlled by medication, the main daily objective is to ensure that her potential in life is reached and that her quality of life is at a premium at all times.

"All we wanted was a 'normal child'; she did not have to be a genius, and she did not have to be a saint or a hero, just 'normal'. But how do you define 'normal', when your 4-year old daughter is diagnosed as having epilepsy? First of all the world drops to somewhere below your knees, you are frightened - no, terrified; what is this going to do to our world? It is all 'who, what, where and why' with a lot of self-pity, recrimination, despair and anger thrown in.

"At the time of diagnosis as parents you are probably in shock, anger and occasionally despair and you need to try and support each other. It is for your own self-interest and your child's to talk to each other about what is going on. It is important though to make sure that when your child is of an age to understand, you do not hide from them what is wrong, explain to them what you know. Seek advice; ask the medics to explain what is happening to your child but make sure they don't 'blind you with science'.

"It is essential that you do not forget to involve any other siblings and relatives, for they have to be made aware of your child's condition, to reduce any fear and anxieties they too may be experiencing. They also need your help and support. Do not have 'secrets' as this causes mistrust. Talk openly about what is happening - then all of you will benefit from this attitude.

"Then it starts: the medication and the tests, the EEG with lots of flashing lights, wires and appearing to give no real result other than to say 'there is a lot of brain activity'.... you already know that. The MRI - the noisy 'polo machine', enough to frighten the wits out of any child - or parent for that matter.

"Then you get the tablets - after having waited three hours in dispensary - and if you have got any sense you read the leaflets and scare the life out of yourself with the side effects! But wait a minute, what about your child - all this is happening to them, not you. You are, in some respects just an observer, dependent on the advice of the medics, in particular your child's consultant. Does the consultant know what they are doing, can you trust them - if so why? At the end of the day what choice do you have? The answer in all probability is …. none.

"You put your faith in the medication hoping that maybe it will help control the seizures and to some point it does. You can even get to the point where you can give your child enough drug therapy to stop the seizures altogether. It can at times seem to be a 'hit and miss' approach; hopefully you will reach a stage where the seizures are controlled, reduced or even fit free. However this may mean the possibility of your child becoming a 'medicated zombie'. You have to strike a balance between the 'medicated zombie' and the 'normal' child, and that is in some respects a harsh decision. When your child is young they may not recognise the fact they have had a seizure so there is no embarrassment factor to them. However, as they grow older and realise post-seizure what has occurred, this can hit them hard and in turn, also you! Yes, a fit can cause embarrassment for both the sufferer and the parents and other carers, but you have to have the strength of personality to overcome this situation, explain to the people around you what is happening and lose your embarrassment - otherwise it won't help the 'sufferer'.

"Don't be frightened to question the medics, they are there to help your child; question the medication as you and your child need to know what, if anything it can or cannot do. Research the books, the internet or anything else, you never know you just might find something that may help you, your child and even the medics! Question everything it is your right to know, but qualify it in that you have to trust the medics because at the end of the day you have to put your faith and your child's medical care in their hands.

"It has been stated that as long as seizures are controlled parents are happy. In our daughter's case, following a change of medication, seizures were indeed controlled; however the downside was to observe a complete person-ality change, with mood swings resulting in violent outbursts and apparent depressive and low esteem periods - gone was our happy-go-lucky teenager. At this stage seizures were a better option for our daughter, the family and her carers. A revision of medication was conducted offering a return to a more settled household, and 'unannounced' seizures.

"The essential component here was that the relationship between our daughter, we as her parents and her physicians had developed and the 'listening factor' was strong with each party informative and supportive to the other.

"As with many chronic diseases and disabilities the psychological factors of anxiety and depression often show themselves through mood swings observed by parents and carers. Physicians need to offer support by recognizing and understanding the need for possible medication change. It can be difficult for parents to know whether the mood swings are part and parcel of their off-springs' medical condition/treatment or the 'terrible twos/threes' etc, or due to the 'hormonal teenager'; in fact, it may just be part of growing up. Unfortunately this is occasionally completely impossible to decipher!

"It is essential that throughout all the trials and tribulations that we face on a daily basis our family life continues in a state of 'abnormal normality'. As a family we take holidays - home and abroad, have days out etc. Obviously greater planning takes place - preferably day-flights to avoid excessive tired-ness (a possible trigger factor for seizures); a series of short walks rather than day-long hikes; at least two carers when our daughter goes swimming. After a while you suddenly realise nothing is impossible when given a little thought. It did however take us a while to gain sufficient confidence to take our daughter to a Premiership football match surrounded by 40,000-plus football supporters. There is no way we will deny, despite the unannounced seizures, our daughter of actually experiencing the excitement of a packed football ground and seeing her beloved team.

"Adopt a common sense approach; watch your child, do not wrap them in cotton wool, as they must be allowed to do what every other child does. They need a sense of freedom, even if it is under a wary (and weary?), watchful eye.

"What do we want? We want our daughter to be fit-free and medication-free. We have previously experienced the joy of our daughter being fit-free and medication-free, one of the best sensations ever only to be followed by the one of the biggest disappointments when the seizures re-commenced. What did we do? We started all over again! It is a long, hard road to travel so start walking ... hopefully we will get there in the end.

"What will we achieve? We do not know; at this stage our daughter is fifteen years old and has learning difficulties and associated medical problems. What is her outlook? It is hard to judge even at this stage in her life. But one thing you can be assured of is we will never give up hope, you never know what will happen. Do what you would do with every other child; enjoy your days out, enjoy your holidays. If you get it wrong, adjust or don't do it again. Give your child a chance - sometimes they surprise you and sometimes you surprise yourself and others. It is not easy, it is not nice, it is frustrating and you will get angry. Do not stop - you have to carry on, what choice do you have? Lock them away and visit them every blue moon as portrayed in the BBC series 'The Lost Prince'? - definitely not. Try to follow a normal routine, at the end of the day they are 'normal' kids with epilepsy; it is you that has to try and be 'normal'.

"The future - who knows? In some respects we are in a state of limbo; our daughter's educational needs have not been met, she has little concept of numbers, she has some short-term memory loss. However she has the person-ality that draws her to all people, young and old alike, so although the future is not altogether rosy, it certainly is not black. For example, within the next few weeks our daughter will be undertaking two weeks work experience in an office environment.

"How will she cope - by herself? We will not be there. Will people recognize that our daughter is having one of her types of seizure as she is sitting staring into space? It will become very apparent when she falls from her chair into a grand mal seizure. Who will cope best? Our daughter; her colleagues, or us as her parents as we travel to collect her – unsure of what to expect when we get there. The public react very differently when seeing someone having a seizure. Some are embarrassed, some frightened, some disgusted and some are very practical and will do whatever it takes to help. It amazes us that many still believe that epilepsy is contagious. It is difficult for people to understand epilepsy and in certain respects it still carries a stigma. We believe that this is due to a lack of public understanding and education, and, to a certain extent, this also extends to the medical fraternity.

"The key priority for us, throughout the good days and the bad (frequent fits), the anger and the frustrations of all parties involved, is to maintain the highest quality of life through love and support for our daughter who has shown us a side of life we would not normally have experienced and by her being able to offer happiness and caring to others despite all the adversities life has bestowed upon her."

Peter and Ida, parents of Elena
(Elena has a cryptogenic partial epilepsy with additional learning difficulties.)

CONCLUSION

Seizure freedom without side-effects from antiepileptic medication is a realistic and achievable goal for the majority of children with epilepsy. For most of these children, seizure freedom is also likely to be sustainable even without the need for life-long antiepileptic medication. Unfortunately, the significant remainder (25% of the entire childhood epilepsy population), will never achieve seizure freedom with our current therapies and even surgical resection of confirmed epileptogenic cerebral cortex cannot guarantee a long-term 'cure' of the epilepsy. The management of these children will inevitably be more difficult and must attempt to balance as optimal as seizure control as possible without any impairment of their ability to learn, play, grow and behave; a balanced discussion is also required on the realistic likelihood of achieving seizure freedom without eliminating all parental hope. Predictably, this is far easier to achieve in theory than in practice and it epitomizes the fact that medical care and delivery is always an art as well as a science.

REFERENCES

Appleton, R.E. (2003). Mortality in paediatric epilepsy. *Arch Dis Child* **88**, 1091-1094.

Arts, W.F., Brouwer, O.F., Peters, A.C., Stroink, H., Peeters, E.A., Schmitz, P.I., van Donselaar, C.A. and Geerts, A.T. (2004). Course and prognosis of childhood epilepsy: 5-year follow-up of the Dutch study of epilepsy in childhood. *Brain* **127**, 1774-1784.

Baker, G.A., Camfield, C., Camfield, P., Cramer, J.A., Elger, C.E., Johnson, A.L., Martins da Silva, A., Meinardi, H., Munari, C., Perucca, E. and Thorbecke, R. (1998). Commission on outcome measurement in epilepsy, 1994-1997: final report. *Epilepsia* **39**, 213-231.

Bourgeois, B.F.D. (1998). Antiepileptic drugs, learning and behaviour in childhood epilepsy. *Epilepsia* **39**, 913-921.

Callenbach, P.M.C., Westendorp, R.G.J., Geerts, A.T., Arts, W.F.M., Peeters, E.A.J., van Donselaar, C.A., Peters, A.C.B., Stroink, H. and Brouwer, O.F. (2001). Mortality risk in children with epilepsy: The Dutch study of epilepsy in childhood. *Pediatrics* **107**, 1259-1263.

Camfield, C.S., Camfield, P.R. and Veugelers, P.J. (2002). Death in children with epilepsy: a population-based study. *Lancet* **359**, 1891-1895.

Dulac, O. (2001). Epileptic encephalopathy. *Epilepsia* **42(Suppl 3)**, S23-S26.

Elger, C.E., Bauer, J., Scherrmann, J. and Widman, G. (1998). Aggravation of focal epileptic seizures by antiepileptic drugs. *Epilepsia* **39(Suppl 3)**, S15-S18.

Engel, J. (2001). A proposed diagnostic scheme for people with epileptic seizures and with epilepsy: report of the ILAE Task Force on Classification and Terminology. *Epilepsia* **42**, 796-803.

Holmes, G.L., Sarkisian, M., Ben-Ari, Y. and Chevassus-Au-Louis, N. (1999). Effects of recurrent seizures in the developing brain. In: Nehlig, A., Motte, J., Moshe, S.L. and Plouin P. (Eds), *Childhood Epilepsies and Brain Development*. John Libbey, London, pp.263-276.

Holmes, G.L. (2002). Over-treatment in children with epilepsy. *Epilepsy Res* **52**, 35-42.

Kemp, A.S. and Sibert, J.R. (1993). Epilepsy in children and the risk of drowning. *Arch Dis Child* **68**, 684-685.

Kirsch, R. and Wirrell, E. (2001). Do cognitively normal children with epilepsy have a higher rate of injury than their non-epileptic peers? *J Child Neurol* **16**, 100-104.

Kwan, P, and Brodie, M.J. (2001). Effectiveness of first antiepileptic drug. *Epilepsia* **42**, 1255-1260.

National Institute for Health and Clinical Excellence. (2004). The epilepsies: the diagnosis and management of the epilepsies in children and young people in primary and secondary care – a quick reference guide. www.nice.org.uk/pdf/CG020childrenquickrefeguide.pdf (published in October 2004).

Schmidt, D., Baumgartner, C. and Löscher, W. (2004). Seizure recurrence after planned discontinuation of antiepileptic drugs in seizure-free patients after epilepsy surgery: a review of current clinical experience. *Epilepsia* **45**, 179-186.

Schmidt, D. and Löscher, W. (2005). Drug resistance in epilepsy: putative neurobiological and clinical mechanisms. *Epilepsia* **46**, 858-877.

Scottish Intercollegiate Guidelines Network. (2005). Diagnosis and management of epilepsies in children and young people. A national clinical guideline. www.sign.ac.uk/pdf/sign81.pdf

Sillanpää, M., Haataja, L. and Shinnar, S. (2004). Perceived impact of childhood-onset epilepsy on quality of life as an adult. *Epilepsia* **45**, 971-977.

Williams, J., Steel, C., Sharp, G.B. *et al.* (2003). Parental anxiety and quality of life in children with epilepsy. *EpilepsyBehav* **4,** 483-486.

Wirrell, E.C., Camfield, P.R., Camfield, C.S., Dooley J.M. and Gordon, KE. (1996). Accidental injury is a serious risk in children with typical absence epilepsy. *Arch Neurol* **53**, 129-132.

Ziegler, A.L., Reinberg, O. and Deonna, T. (1994). Epilepsy and accidents: what is the risk in children? *Arch Ped* **1**, 801-805.

Seizure Freedom: Clinical, Research and Quality of Life Perspectives
Edited by Michael R. Trimble
© 2006 Clarius Press Ltd

7

Sudden Unexpected
Death in Epilepsy

LINA NASHEF

*King's College Hospital,
London, UK*

INTRODUCTION

It is appropriate that SUDEP, or sudden death in epilepsy, the single most important category of epilepsy- related deaths, is included in a textbook on seizure freedom, and in this chapter, I hope to present evidence that supports this statement. Sudden death in epilepsy is now well recognised. It is studied, debated and, to some extent, feared. It is also mourned. Fortunately, it is relatively infrequent. In recent years, there has been much debate as to whether information on SUDEP should be communicated to patients and carers. Those who believe that the risk of SUDEP cannot be influenced see potential harm, and little value, in raising this issue for people with epilepsy who already have much to contend with. Others, believing or hoping that some of these deaths may be preventable, hold the opposite view. Some, like Epilepsy Bereaved, the UK-based self-help group (www.SUDEP.org), also advocate the patients' right to know. Patients, however, seek and have access to many resources, and the physician's role is perhaps more that of individualising the risk for each patient and putting it in perspective. In this era of widely available information, it may be that the debate, of whether to inform or not, will become redundant. Nevertheless, it has value in encouraging us to examine the evidence.

No one disputes the risks associated with uncontrolled epileptic seizures. Risk of accidental injury, burns and drowning are well recognised and are exposure-dependent. There is also a risk to life and of associated morbidity with status epilepticus. Although some individuals are much more susceptible than others, status epilepticus, in chronic epilepsy, is to a certain extent preventable, by avoiding abrupt medication changes, adherence to treatment and by early treatment of escalating seizures or prolonged convulsions. It is unknown to what extent sudden death in epilepsy is preventable. At one extreme, SUDEP is viewed as a mystery we do not begin to understand and thus cannot prevent, associated with biological factors we have no control over. At the other extreme, it is considered largely a seizure-related event which may be avoided by preventing seizures, by ensuring an optimal response when seizures occur and by improving service provision for those with epilepsy. The expert panel review of epilepsy-related deaths, including SUDEP, identified in the UK National Sentinel Audit, considered that 39% of adult epilepsy-related deaths were potentially or probably avoidable (www.nice.org.uk, May 2002). So what is the evidence? This chapter will address the relationship between SUDEP and epileptic seizures, outline risk factors identified so far and discuss theories regarding mechanisms, before returning to the issue of information provision.

DEFINITIONS

Unexpected sudden deaths occur in otherwise well individuals with epilepsy in benign circumstances with no cause found at autopsy. The following pragmatic definition has the advantage of being workable:

Sudden, unexpected witnessed or unwitnessed, non-traumatic, and non-drowning death in patients with epilepsy with or without evidence for a seizure and excluding documented status epilepticus where post-mortem examination does not reveal a structural or toxicological cause for death (Nashef, 1997).

Not everyone agrees with the above definition, some choosing to exclude cases with a known epileptic seizure from the category of SUDEP. The main reason for favouring this inclusive definition relates to the difficulty in differentiating, with any certainty, seizure-related deaths from those occurring in the absence of an epileptic seizure, particularly when the death is unwitnessed. It must be stressed that SUDEP, is not a condition, cause or mechanism. It is simply a convenient category in which to classify such deaths. The above definition refers to *definite* SUDEP cases. However, regrettably, autopsy is not always performed. For the purpose of epidemiological studies, sudden death occurring in benign circumstances with no known competing cause for death, is classified as *probable* SUDEP. Other categories are possible SUDEP, where there is a competing cause, or *not SUDEP* with a clear cause of death established (Annegers, 1997).

It can perhaps be argued that the above approach is not inclusive enough, and that we also need broader categories. Issues for further study and internal and external comparisons in relation to operational definitions are discussed by Hauser (1997). By not considering cases with co-existing predisposing pathology, we cannot assess the increased risk when this combines with uncontrolled epilepsy. Two illustrative cases, highlight this (Nashef *et al.*, 1998). In both, witnesses described terminal habitual epileptic seizures; post-mortem examination showed significant ischaemic heart disease, which the pathologist reasonably considered as the cause of death. Such cases are appropriately excluded from the pure category of SUDEP, despite the deaths being clearly related to epileptic seizures. Studies, however, should also address the, potentially more than additive, excess risk of sudden death in individuals with epilepsy who have other pathologies. This is particularly relevant in children with multiple handicap and in the elderly. It may also be relevant in the case of a convulsive seizure associated with head injury or intoxication.

PROFILE OF SUDEP VICTIMS AND RELATION TO EPILEPTIC SEIZURES

The majority of SUDEP cases are unwitnessed and most are found dead in bed having been well the evening before. Birnbach and colleagues (1991), in an early case-control study, reported an association with convulsive seizures. One case report of a documented SUDEP case occurred in a video telemetry unit during a secondary generalized epileptic seizure (Bird *et al.*, 1997), an informative case as death was preceded by (post)-ictal generalised EEG flattening. In an unwitnessed case, circumstances that suggest, but do not prove, an epileptic seizure include fresh tongue, cheek or lip biting, secretions, incontinence, disrupted environment or bedding, fall off the bed or timing and triggers as per habitual seizures. A very useful study by Ulrich and Maxeiner (2003) retrospectively looked at tongue bite marks in deaths of 105 individuals with a known history of epilepsy compared to a control group of 107 with sudden cardiac death. Marks were only present in 2% of the control group and there was no association with attempted resuscitation. Among the epilepsy group, tongue bite marks were seen in 21% of the whole group and in 64% of those with "observed death during seizure", significantly more than the control group. Among 41 of 70 'natural' deaths in the epilepsy group, an exact cause was not ascertainable. They categorised 29 of these as SUDEP of whom 17 showed bite marks as did half of the remaining 12 cases. Head injuries were reported in 41% of the epilepsy group, and in 73% of those with "observed death during seizure". They concluded that the "presence of fresh bite marks of the tongue, according to histological findings, is a useful sign for the assignment of death to an epileptic seizure and especially for death during acute convulsion".

It is clear that the absence of suggestive evidence, including tongue bite, does not exclude a terminal epileptic event. Indirect evidence suggests that SUDEP is frequently a peri-ictal event. The proportion of witnessed cases vary. These have been summarized as reported occurring in 7–38% of the total, with between one third and 100% of those witnessed related to convulsions (Langan *et al.*, 2000). These authors reported terminal convulsions amongst 12/15 witnessed SUDEP cases, amongst the first 135 ascertained for a large UK case-control study. An older study addressed circumstances of death based on detailed interviews of bereaved relatives or partners of 26 SUDEP victims, including two witnessed with terminal convulsions (Nashef *et al.*, 1998). Among the remaining 24 unwitnessed cases, there was evidence suggestive of an epileptic seizure in 21. The evidence varied from physical evidence, such as tongue or mouth bites, incontinence, disruption of environment and falls off the bed to circumstantial evidence such as timing and / or circumstances of habitual seizures. The latter included an untreated youth with pure photosensitive epilepsy found dead by a VDU screen, a reported trigger for all previous convulsions. Signs of preceding seizures were also reported in 67% in a Norwegian case-control study of 42 SUDEP cases (Kloster *et al.*, 1999).

It is, however, difficult to compare studies in this regard; the information available differs between studies, not all studies list the evidence found and most studies do not seek detailed information. The UK case-control study of a final total of 154 SUDEP cases also reported evidence for a seizure in the majority (Langan *et al.*, 2005). Finally, observations from case-control studies, discussed further below, report a higher relative risk in people with more frequent seizures and in those with a history of generalised convulsive seizures.

In conclusion, the majority of SUDEP cases are likely to be related to a convulsive epileptic seizure occurring close to the time of death, but this can only account for part of the evidence. Why some individuals are more at risk than others, with a similar profile, is still not yet well understood and other risk factors need to be considered. Some individuals may be more at risk because of social factors, life-style, sub-optimal management and lack of adherence to treatment. Others have additional biological susceptibilities.

Older descriptive cohorts provide a profile of those at risk and suggest potential risk factors for study. Influential early observational studies from Leestma and colleagues (1989) from the Office of the Medical Examiner of Cook County (Chicago) drew attention to SUDEP. The profile of those more at risk following their prospective study was of black males, averaging 35 years of age, with infrequent generalised seizures, structural brain lesion, who tended to abuse alcohol and have poor compliance. This profile, likely to have been influenced by local factors, cannot but raise the possibility that some of those deaths were avoidable.

In general, factors emerging from descriptive studies include youth, male sex, remote symptomatic epilepsy, structural findings on neuropathology, severe epilepsy, unwitnessed seizures, alcohol abuse, abnormal EEGs with epileptiform changes and greater variations, mental handicap, psychotropic medication, African-Americans, lack of adherence to treatment, abrupt medication changes and low AED levels. Factors that have been shown to be associated with an increased or decreased risk of SUDEP in case-control studies are discussed later.

SUDEP Incidence

The background risk of sudden death in the general population is around 0.05-0.1/1000 for those under 45 years of age and 3/1000 if older (Annegers, 1997). Rates of SUDEP in incidence studies in various cohorts have been reviewed (Tomson et al., 2005; Stollberger and Finsterer, 2004; O'Donoghue and Sander, 1997). Most cohorts are selected. Large population based studies are difficult to achieve. A population based study from Rochester, USA, with 9 SUDEP cases observed a SUDEP rate of 0.35/1000 person-years (Ficker et al., 1998). A multicentre unselected hospital series from the USA reported a rate of 1.21/1000 (Walczak et al., 2001). The rate is extremely low in new onset incidence cases, and in those with controlled epilepsy (Lhatoo et al., 2001; MRC AED Withdrawal Study Group, 1991). Broadly speaking, among prevalent cases, the rate is less than 1:1000 person years of follow-up in the community and of the order of 1:250/year in special cohorts or those seen in specialist services. It is higher still in intractable series considered for epilepsy surgery (Dasheiff, 1991).

The risks quoted above relate to adults. In the elderly, sudden death as defined above is difficult to study, as competing co-morbidity is more likely and attribution is difficult. Furthermore, excess mortality due to epilepsy is likely to be lost within much higher death rates in general. SUDEP is also known to occur in children and has been reported in both symptomatic and idiopathic epilepsies, much more commonly in the former (Harvey et al., 1993; Sillanpää et al., 1998; Donner et al., 2001; Camfield et al., 2002; Weber et al., 2005). Overall it is thought to be 'rare', although more likely to be observed in specialised units. Mortality is considered more often related to the underlying neurological disorder or associated deficit rather than to epileptic seizures. Sillanpaa's long term study, which uses different definitions, separating deaths in a seizure from SUDEP, observed an overall mean age of death of 18.6 years (range of 1-41), suggesting a greater risk as children became young adults.

What is very much lacking are long term prospective studies of mortality and SUDEP rates in specific syndromes. A differential SUDEP rate, in different syndromes, with similar seizure types, may provide further clues about mechanisms. Another important area is how medical, surgical or social intervention can influence the rate of SUDEP. Double blind randomised placebo controlled studies addressing whether treatment reduces SUDEP rates are evidently unethical! The effect of intervention on SUDEP risk can, therefore, only be gleaned from indirect evidence.

SUDEP and surgical treatment

Patients treated with Vagus Nerve Stimulation, particularly in the first few years after it was introduced, generally had severe epilepsy. A sudden death rate of 4.5/1000 for definite/probable SUDEP (6:1000 if possible cases were included) was observed (Annegers et al., 1998). This is comparable to that expected in an intractable cohort. Interestingly this rate seemed to decrease with longer follow-up (Annegers et al., 2000) but this has not been studied further. The use of this treatment has escalated in recent years and further studies are both feasible and necessary.

A number of studies address mortality including SUDEP rates following epilepsy surgery (Ryvlin and Kahane, 2003). Two general observations can be made at the outset. As already stated, those undergoing pre-surgical evaluation appear to be at particularly high risk, as are patients evaluated for surgery but not operated on (Vickrey et al., 1995; Vickrey, 1997). Furthermore, overall long-term mortality remains elevated following surgery for epilepsy with observed epilepsy related deaths due to a variety of causes, including suicide, status epileptics, accidental deaths and SUDEP (Jensen, 1975; Taylor and Marsh, 1977; Hennessy et al., 1999; Salanova et al., 2002; Nilsson et al., 2003; Stavem and Guldvog, 2005; Sperling et al., 1999; 2005). At face value, it appears that successful surgery is associated with a lower mortality (Vickrey et al., 1995; Vickrey, 1997; Salanova et al., 2002; Sperling et al., 1999; 2005) In two studies, none of the SUDEP cases were seizure- free (Sperling et al., 2005; Nilsson et al., 2003). It is likely that successful epilepsy surgery results in a lower risk. However, an additional interpretation, which is also likely, is that those with successful surgery differ biologically from the failed or rejected surgery groups. In support of this hypothesis, are the results of a study which showed a difference in pre-operative heart rate variability (HRV) between patients with good and poor outcome of surgery for temporal lobe epilepsy (Persson et al., 2005). An earlier study showed differences in pre-surgical HRV patterns between poor candidates for epilepsy surgery and those with excellent outcome of temporal lobe resection (Frysinger et al., 1993). Hilz and colleagues (2003) also reported differences in HRV between patients who became seizure free and those with persistent seizures.

Risk factors in case-control studies

Certain risk factors have been shown to be associated with SUDEP in case-control studies. These studies have different methodologies and are not directly comparable. Some studies, for example, only include patients on long term treatment for epilepsy or in specified age ranges. Not all studies are nested and not all addressed the same variables. Control groups in particular vary and include alive patients known to have epilepsy or patients with epilepsy who died of other causes, the latter may be from another at-risk group and may have more severe epilepsy, which could bias analysis of risk factors. SUDEP cases and controls are identified from a variety of sources and this can result in different data being available. Negative results should not be taken to exclude an association; even studies with good numbers of SUDEP cases may have reduced power in relation to certain variables because of incomplete data.

Some case-control studies with a reasonable number of SUDEP cases are summarised here and discussed further below:

Norwegian study

Kloster and Engelskjon (1999) reported on a cohort of 42 SUDEP cases from Norway, identified from an outpatient cohort at a tertiary referral centre. Only those who had had post-mortem examination were considered, 61 deaths having been excluded. Deaths with a verifiable cause for death served as controls. The profile of SUDEP cases was similar to other studies. A high seizure frequency was observed in both cases and controls. The study showed a significant association with the prone position in SUDEP cases. Hyponatraemia was observed in two SUDEP cases.

Swedish Study

Nilsson and colleagues (1999) reported on 57 hospital based SUDEP cases, aged 15-70, among whom 52 had undergone post-mortem examination, four others had died in association with witnessed seizures in hospital and the fifth died suddenly in the community. Deaths and living age and sex-matched controls were identified from a cohort of cases admitted to and discharged from all hospitals in the County of Stockholm. A major aim of the study was comparing drug treatment, and only cases who had been treated with one of three major anti-epileptic drugs (AEDs), namely phenytoin, carbamazepine or valproate, for a year or more were included. Positive associations included: More frequent seizures [RR=10.16 (95% CI 2.94-35.18) more than 50 seizures/year vs. 2]; epilepsy type with a lower risk in symptomatic focal vs. idiopathic generalised epilepsy, but the numbers here were small; epilepsy age of onset [RR= 7.72 (95% CI 2.13-27.96) for age 0-15 years vs. 45 years]; polytherapy [RR = 9.89 (95% CI 3.20-30.60) 3 AED's vs. monotherapy]; and frequent medication changes [RR = 6.08 (95% CI 1.99-18.56) for 3-5 changes/year vs. none].

Minneapolis US Study

Walczak and colleagues (2001) reported on a case-control study of 20 SUDEP cases. Although SUDEP cases were fewer than the other studies listed here, the study included an unselected cohort of 4,578 patients identified from three epilepsy centres and followed up prospectively for 16,463 patient years, thus providing data on incidence. Controls were living cases recruited from the same cohort. The following associations were observed: IQ less than 70 vs IQ greater than 79 [OR=5 (95% CI 1.3-19.3)]; more than two AEDs vs. 0-2 [OR=4.0 (95% CI 1.4-11.7)]; tonic clonic seizures (GTCS) in the past year [1-3 GTCS, OR 2.4 (95% CI 1.8-30.5); more than three GTCS [OR 8.1 (95% CI 2.2-30.0)]; more than 50 seizures/month [OR=11.5 (95%CI 1.3-99.3)].

UK study

This study includes the largest SUDEP cases to date. Langan and colleagues (2005) reported on 154 SUDEP cases, aged 16-50, identified through coroners, neurologists and through the self help group Epilepsy Bereaved. Controls were age matched living epilepsy patients identified from general practice records in the same geographical area as SUDEP cases. The study was not nested. The level of information available varied with some subjects and controls. Significant associations with an increased risk of SUDEP included history of GTCS [OR = 13.8 (95% CI 6.6-29.1)]; history of GTCS in the last three months [OR= 13.8 (95% CI 6.6-29.1)]; more than four AEDs ever taken compared to 1-2 [OR=3.1 (95% CI 1.4-7)]; having never taken AEDs [OR 21.7 (95% CI 4.4-106)]; and prescription of carbamazepine [OR= 2 (95% CI 1.1-3.8)]. Interestingly, an association with a protective effect was observed with sharing a bedroom with an individual capable of giving assis-tance [OR= 0.4 (95% CI 0.2-0.8)] and the use of listening devices [OR= 0.1 (95% CI 0.0-0.3)].

SUDEP and anti-epileptic drugs

It may be useful to discuss evidence related to AEDs and SUDEP. Of note is that SUDEP was observed and documented well before the era of modern AED therapy. Medications taken by SUDEP victims in various cohorts studied appear to reflect prescribing practices. Nevertheless, factors relating to AED treatment are potentially very important, as these are amenable to manipulation in routine medical management. Such factors include individual drug effects, drug levels, adherence to treatment, the effect of abrupt withdrawal and polytherapy.

The Swedish study, which only included SUDEP cases with treated epilepsy, identified polytherapy and frequent medication changes, among others, as independent risk factors for SUDEP. These risk factors are likely to be surrogate markers for epilepsy severity. Theoretically, however, these factors could make SUDEP more likely. Frequent or abrupt medication changes, can result in instability of the epilepsy or of the autonomic nervous system. AED therapy, including polytherapy, could also affect post-ictal respiratory depression or predispose to cardiac arrhythmias. The effect of medication choice, medication changes or polytherapy on modifying seizure severity including the post-ictal phase, as opposed to seizure type or frequency, is not adequately studied; yet, anecdotally, such an effect is familiar to practicing clinicians and is often reported by carers.

The Swedish group also investigated the potential of AEDs to inhibit the cardiac rapid delayed rectifier potassium ion current (I_{Kr}). Other drugs known to have such an effect can be proarrhythmic and their clinical use associated with sudden unexpected death. Phenytoin, phenobarbital and lamotrigine have the potential to inhibit the I_{Kr} channel at potentially clinically relevant concentrations, while the blocking effect of carbamazepine, topiramate and gabapentin occurred at concentrations outside those associated with a clinical effect (Danielsson et al., 2003; 2005).

HRV can provide a measure of autonomic cardiac control and reduced HRV has been shown to predict sudden death in conditions other than epilepsy The high frequency band on spectral analysis of HRV reflects parasympathetic activity and low frequency mainly sympathetic activity. Many studies have shown reduced HRV in epilepsy in adults and children, mainly in those with partial epilepsy including those with temporal lobe epilepsy and on carbamazepine, although little is known of the effect of other antiepileptic drugs. Changes in HRV have also been reported after abrupt withdrawal of carbamazepine or phenytoin (Pomeranz et al., 1985; Takase et al., 1992; Bigger et al., 1993; Kenebäck et al., 1997; Massetani et al., 1997; Tomson et al., 1998; Ansakorpi et al., 2000; Hennessy et al., 2001; Yang et al., 2001; Ferri et al., 2002; Ansakorpi et al., 2002; Persson et al., 2003; Eppinger et al., 2004; Ronkainen et al., 2005; Evrengul et al., 2005).

The UK study did not confirm polytherapy as a risk factor. The study, however, reported an increased risk in association with the total number of AEDs ever taken, most likely reflecting on the intractability of the epilepsy. The same study found untreated epilepsy to be a significant risk factor. This is an important observation, which, along with the association of SUDEP with convulsive seizures, supports active treatment of epilepsy with AEDs. Risks associated with treatment interventions, surgical or medical, are well recognised, including the potential to worsen seizure frequency. The balance between risk and benefit, however, favours appropriate AED treatment and the prevention of convulsive seizures.

Studies on adherence to treatment are contradictory, some supporting treatment non-adherence as a risk factor, others not (Bowerman *et al.*, 1978; Lund *et al.*, 1985; Opeskin *et al.*, 1999; George *et al.*, 1998). This is not surprising in view of inevitable methodological limitations. Details on medication taken, rather than prescribed, in the few days preceding death, often cannot be reliably ascertained. Post-mortem AED blood levels can be unreliable (Tomson *et al.*, 1998), and levels below the usual quoted ranges are often therapeutic; absolute levels may be less important than changes in level from usual maintenance; comparisons are made difficult because of the importance of timing in relation to samples taken and degradation of post-mortem samples. An interesting recent study from Cardiff, UK measured AED levels in sequential one-centimeter hair segment samples, corrected for wash-out effects. A limitation of the technique is that results do not reflect AED changes immediately before death. The study showed greater coefficient of variation in SUDEP cases than in three other cohorts studied: an epilepsy cohort dying of other known causes, an outpatient cohort and a residential cohort, with the latter showing the lowest variation. The difference, as far as the authors could ascertain, was not attributable to prescribed medication changes (Williams *et al.*, 2006). This study suggests that non-adherence to treatment may indeed be a significant risk factor.

The question as to whether specific AEDs are associated with a higher risk of SUDEP has been raised. Timmings and colleagues (Timmings, 1998) reported that carbamazepine was disproportionately represented in patients suffering SUDEP. Further analysis of the Swedish study (Nilsson *et al.*, 2001) suggested an increased risk, in patients with frequent dose changes and polytherapy, with carbamazepine levels greater than the commonly quoted target range, this being the case in only six cases. The UK study showed a small excess risk with carbamazepine treatment just reaching significance. Rare cases of heart block secondary to carbamazepine have been reported and carbamazepine affects HRV. Nevertheless, the relevance of this association to the majority of people with epilepsy is uncertain; it is likely that those with more severe seizures were prescribed carbamazepine, at higher doses, as it is has been a main-stay of treatment in Europe in the 1980s and 1990s. AED treatment, however, needs to be appropriate to the epilepsy syndrome. In one study, some SUDEP cases on carbamazepine had uncontrolled idiopathic generalised epilepsy, where a broad spectrum medication may have had better success (Nashef *et al.*, 1998). The US Minneapolis study did not identify an association with any particular AED. In a recent review, Walczak (2003) reasonably argues that, on current evidence, there is no strong reason to avoid any particular AED. He stressed the importance of preventing tonic-clonic seizures with as few AEDs as necessary to achieve complete control.

MECHANISMS

Pathological studies, by definition, do not reveal a cause of death. This suggests that the terminal event is likely to be due to functional, not structural, disturbances. The monitored SUDEP case at a telemetry unit, where death occurred during a secondarily generalised tonic clonic seizure, has already been referred to. It is uncertain how often the observed EEG flattening, which presumably reflects cerebral shutdown, occurs. Death was presumably mediated initially through respiratory insufficiency as a persistent perfusion pulse artefact, recorded through an intracranial electrode, was noted for a further 120 seconds after EEG flattening (Bird *et al.*, 1997). The EEG pattern while recognized has not been studied in a systematic manner. It is likely to be rare.

Post-mortem examination in SUDEP cases may reveal tongue bites or petechial haemorrhages, a non-specific finding in hypoxia and increased venous pressure. Pulmonary oedema is very frequently noted in addition to other organ congestion. Death, although sudden, may not be instantaneous in all cases with a study of the neuropathology in SUDEP cases showing microscopic evidence of hypoxic change in a small proportion of cases (Thom, 1997). Routine autopsies in SUDEP cases, by definition, do not reveal a cardiac, or other cause, for death. Two studies reported on specialised cardiac pathology (Natelson *et al.*, 1998; Opeskin *et al.*, 2000) with the changes reported of uncertain significance. Perivascular and interstitial cardiac fibrosis, mainly sub-endocardial, was found in four SUDEP cases and myocyte vacuolization in a fifth but not in the control group. In another study, morphological abnormalities of the cardiac conduction system were observed in 4/10 SUDEP cases, with a similar finding in 6/10 of the control group. This does not exclude these changes contributing to death in either group.

Respiratory mechanisms

Respiratory changes frequently occur in seizures with well-documented central and obstructive apnoea, excess bronchial and oral secretions, pulmonary oedema and hypoxia (Stollberger and Finsterer, 2004; Nashef, 2004). Pulmonary oedema is present in a large majority of SUDEP cases. Central apnoea can occur secondary to the ictal discharge or post-ictally. In a sheep model of ictal sudden death, the animals that died were those with a greater rise in pulmonary vascular pressure and hypoventilation. When airway obstruction was excluded in a second study of tracheostomised sheep, central apnoea and hypoventilation were observed in all animals, causing or contributing to death in two. A third animal developed heart failure with significant pathological cardiac ischaemic changes (Johnston *et al.*, 1995; 1997). These studies support an important role for ictal apnoea/hypoventilation.

A number of possible reasons may be put forward to explain the observation that most unwitnessed SUDEP deaths occur in bed, presumably during sleep. Nocturnal seizures may differ pathophysiologically; they may be associated with an increase in vagal tone or other sleep-induced cardiac arrhythmias or more marked respiratory depression. The lack of assistance at the time of the terminal event is likely to be important. The Norwegian case-control study found a significant difference in the position in which the body was found compared to that expected, with 71% prone and only 4% supine. In the study of circumstances (Nashef *et al.*, 1998), in 11 of 26 SUDEP cases, the body was found in a position which predisposed to respiratory obstruction. In another study of a cohort of residential school children with epilepsy and other disability, where children were monitored at night by awake staff aided by a continuous nocturnal sound monitoring system, 14 SUDEP cases occurred during the period of study and all took place while the children were away from school (Nashef *et al.*, 1995). Finally, the use of listening devices or sharing the room with someone capable of giving assistance, was associated with a reduced risk in the UK case-control study. The evidence that supervision within the community provides some protection favours an important primary role for respiratory factors which can be alleviated by relatively unskilled intervention such as adjusting position, ensuring an adequate airway and perhaps physically stimulating respiration.

Cardiac mechanisms

Studies on post-mortem cardiac pathology have already been referred to, as was the sheep investigation, in the animal model of sudden death, which developed heart failure with significant pathological cardiac ischaemic changes. Primary or secondary cardiac mechanisms are likely to be important through a number of possible mechanisms, although routine inter-ictal ECG recordings in people with epilepsy have a low diagnostic yield. ECG changes, both of rhythm or repolarization, are documented during seizures, the most common observed change being sinus tachycardia; malignant tachy-arrhythmias are relatively rare. Sinus bradycardia and / or arrest, while still infrequent, are more often documented (Stollberger and Finsterer, 2004). A study from Germany observed ictal cardiac asystole in only 5/1,244 inpatients undergoing prolonged EEG-video recording (Rocamora *et al.*, 2003). Another study looked at cardiac rhythm changes in a highly selected patient group with intractable epilepsy over prolonged periods using an implantable device. Episodes of sinus arrest, for which cardiac pacing was carried out, were recorded in four of 19 patients (Rugg-Gunn *et al.*, 2004). Larger similar studies in different patients groups are needed. The indications for pacing and its potential to prevent seizure-associated syncope and sudden death remain to be established.

Malignant cardiac tachy/brady-arrhythmias or failure may occur secondary to the ictal discharge and/or apnoea/hypoxia. The question also arises as to whether some individuals with epilepsy may have a co-existing 'mild' susceptibility to epilepsy and to sudden cardiac death which can manifest in the presence of uncontrolled seizures and which, theoretically, can be modified by AEDs. Such a susceptibility could be either acquired or genetic. The latter could be inherited as a complex trait through, for example, cardiac conduction/ion channel disorders. This may be unrelated to the epilepsy, or alternatively, in theory, the same genetic variants may confer increased susceptibility to both epilepsy and to sudden cardiac death. Both are paroxysmal conditions in which similar disorders of ion channels, which can be co-expressed in the brain and heart, are causally implicated. It should be noted that inherited susceptibility to arrhythmias can predispose to both bradycardia and tachyarrhythmias. While a family history of cardiac death is not found in SUDEP cases, this does not exclude the possibility of mild complexly inherited susceptibility traits becoming manifest in the presence of uncontrolled epilepsy.

There may be lessons in this context from the study of Sudden Infant Death Syndrome (SIDS). The realisation of the importance of respiratory mechanisms at a vulnerable stage in development of the infant let to dramatic success in reducing the incidence of SIDS, simply by recommending the supine rather than the prone position (Dwyer *et al.*, 1991). Meanwhile, recognising that SIDS was likely to be multifactorial, Schwartz and colleagues prospectively tested their hypothesis that QT interval prolongation may be relevant to SIDS by increasing the risk of life-threatening ventricular arrhythmias. They recorded early electrocardiograms in 34,442 newborns; by one year there were 34 deaths of whom 24 were SIDS cases. The latter had a longer corrected QT interval (QTc) than survivors (mean [+/-SD], 435+/-45 vs. 400+/–20 msec, P<0.01) or infants dying of other causes (393+/–24 msec, P<0.05). Twelve of 24 SIDS victims, but none of the other infants, had a prolonged QTc greater than 440 msec. The odds ratio for SIDS in infants with a prolonged QTc was 41.3 (95% CI 17.3-98.4) (Schwartz *et al.*, 1998) Later, they reported a sporadic SCN5A mutation in a near miss SIDS case and there have been other reports of long QT genetic defects since. The exact contribution of genetic susceptibility to cardiac arrhythmia and SIDS is still to be defined as well as the relationship between this and respiratory factors, but direct causation has been proved in some cases of SIDS as well as stillbirths.

CONCLUSIONS

SUDEP is a significant category of death amongst patients with chronic active epilepsy, particularly in association with convulsive seizures. Information on relative risk in different syndromes is lacking and we need to seek a better understanding of mechanisms. We also need to be better able to identify at risk individuals.

In relation to information provision, at present, there is a divergence, at least in the UK, between what guidelines and patient groups advocate and what is currently practiced. In a study by Morton and colleagues (2006), 82% of UK specialist neurologists, of whom 31% stated a special interest in epilepsy, responded to a questionnaire. Five per cent reported that they discussed SUDEP with all patients, 26% with a majority, 61% with a few and 7.5% with none. Often the discussion was patient led. The authors noted that there were no studies on the impact of telling patients about SUDEP. Their study showed that practice was out of tune with guidelines from medical opinion leaders and patient advocates maintaining that people be given as much information as possible. Such guidelines, they felt, could deny the patient's right not to know and undermine the physician's ability to treat patients as individuals.

On the basis of current evidence, with the aim of preventing some SUDEP cases, the focus in management is on prevention of generalised seizures and on optimising the response to seizures. Best management requires not only expert medical intervention, but also self-management with an understanding by the patient of the principles of AED use and of the importance of avoiding seizure triggers. An optimal response to seizures requires the presence of someone capable of giving assistance and this impinges on hard-won independence. Patients vary as to the level of risk they wish to take, be it in opting to try different or newly licensed AEDs, in considering surgical treatment, in considering independent living, or, if controlled, in choosing to withdraw medication. It is not possible for people to make such decisions without being aware of the risks associated with epilepsy, including SUDEP. While, in my view, there is sufficient evidence to suggest that some SUDEP deaths are potentially preventable, it is not possible to estimate the proportion, nor indeed to give more than broad estimates of risk in individual cases. My practice is to make sure that the patient is informed that there are potentially avoidable risks, including to life, associated with seizures and to tailor individual discussion further depending on individual and social circumstances, treatment options under consideration and the patient's wishes.

REFERENCES

Ansakorpi, H., Korpelainen, J.T., Suominen, K. *et al.* (2000). Interictal cardiovascular autonomic responses in patients with temporal lobe epilepsy. *Epilepsia* **41**, 42-47.

Ansakorpi, H., Korpelainen, J.T., Huikuri, H.V. *et al.* (2002). Heart rate dynamics in refractory and well controlled temporal lobe epilepsy. *J Neurol Neurosurg Psychiatry* **72**, 26-30.

Annegers, J.F. (1997). United States perspective on definitions and classification Epilepsy & Sudden Death. *Epilepsia* **38(Suppl 11)**, S9-S12.

Annegers, J.F., Coan, S.P., Hauser, W.A., Leestma, J., Duffell, W. and Tavern, B. (1998). Epilepsy, vagal nerve stimulation by the NCP System, mortality and sudden unexpected unexplained death. *Epilepsia* **39**, 206-212.

Annegers, J.F., Coan, S.P., Hauser, W.A. and Leestma, J. (2000). Epilepsy, vagal nerve stimulation by the NCP system, all-cause mortality, and sudden, unexpected, unexplained death. *Epilepsia* **41**, 549-553.

Bigger, J.T. Jr., Fleiss, J.L., Rolnitzky, L.M. *et al.* (1993). Frequency domain measures of heart period variability to assess risk late after myocardial infarction. *J Am Coll Cardiol* **21**, 729-736.

Birnbach, C.D., Wilensky, A.J. and Dodrill, C.B. (1991). Predictors of early mortality and sudden death in epilepsy. A multidisciplinary approach. *J Epilepsy* **4**, 11-17.

Bird, J.M., Dembny, K.A.T., Sandeman, D. and Butler, S. (1997). Sudden unexplained death in epilepsy: an intracranially monitored case. *Epilepsia* **38 (Suppl 11)**, S52-S56.

Bowerman, D.L., Levisky, J.A., Urich, R.W. and Wittenberg, P.H. (1978). Premature deaths in persons with seizure disorders – Sub-therapeutic levels of anticonvulsant drugs in post-mortem blood specimens. *J Forensic Sc* **23**, 522-526.

Camfield, C.S., Camfield, P.R. and Veugelers, P.J. (2002). Death in children with epilepsy: a population-based study. *Lancet*. **359**, 1891-1895.

Danielsson, B.R., Lansdell, K., Patmore, L. and Tomson, T. (2003). Phenytoin and phenobarbital inhibit human hERG potassium channels. *Epilepsy Res* **55**, 147-157.

Danielsson, B.R., Lansdell, K., Patmore, L. and Tomson, T. (2005). Effects of the antiepileptic drugs lamotrigine, topiramate and gabapentin on hERG potassium currents. *Epilepsy Res* **63**, 17-25.

Dasheiff, R.M. (1991). Sudden unexpected death in epilepsy: a series from an epilepsy surgery program and speculation on the relationship to sudden cardiac death. *J Clin Neurophysiol* **8**, 216-222.

Donner, E.J., Smith, C.R. and Snead, O.C. (2001). Sudden unexplained death in children with epilepsy. *Neurology* **57**, 430-434.

Dwyer, T., Ponsonby, A.L., Newman, N.M. and Gibbons, L.E. (1991). Prospective cohort study of prone sleeping position and sudden infant death syndrome. *Lancet* **337**, 1244-1247.

Eppinger, N., Shaumann, R., Jokeit, H., *et al.* (2004). Reduced heart rate variability (HRV) in victims of sudden death in epilepsy (SUDEP). *Epilepsia* **45 (Suppl 3)**, S65.

Evrengul, H., Tanriverdi, H., Dursunoglu, D., Kaftan, A., Kuru, O. and Kilic, M. (2005) Time and frequence domain analyses of heart rate variability in patients with epilepsy. *Epilepsy Res* **63**, 131-139.

Ferri, R., Curzi-Dascalova, L., Arzimanoglou, A., Bourgeois, M., Beaud, C., Lahorgue Nunes, M., Elia, M., Musumeci, S.O. and Tripodi, M. (2002). Heart rate variability during sleep in children with partial epilepsy. *J Sleep Res* **11**, 153-160.

Ficker, D.M., So, E.L., Annegers, J.F., O'Brien, P.C., Cascino, G.D. and Belau, P.G. (1998). Population-based study of the incidence of sudden unexplained death in epilepsy. *Neurology* **51**, 1270-1274.

Frysinger, R.C., Engel, J. and Harper, R.M. (1993). Interictal heart rate patterns in partial seizure disorders. *Neurology* **43**, 2136-2139.

George, J.R. and Davis, G.G. (1998). Comparison of anti-epileptic drug levels in different cases of sudden death. *J Forensic Sci.* **43**, 598-603.

Harvey, A.S., Nolan, T. and Carlin, J.B. (1993). Community-based study of mortality in children with epilepsy. *Epilepsia* **34**, 597-603.

Hauser, W.A. (1997). Sudden Unexpected Death in Epilepsy: Issues for further study. *Epilepsy* **38 (Suppl 11)**, S26-S29.

Hennessy, M.J., Langan, Y., Elwes, R.D. *et al.* (1999). A study of mortality after temporal lobe epilepsy surgery. *Neurology* **53**, 1276-1283.

Hennessy, M.J., Tighe, M.G., Binnie, C.D. and Nashef, L. (2001). Sudden withdrawal of carbamazepine increases cardiac sympathetic activity in sleep. *Neurology* **57**, 1650-1654.

Hilz, M.J., Platsch, G., Druschky, K. *et al.* (2003). Outcome of epilepsy surgery correlates with sympathetic modulation and neuroimaging of the heart. *J Neurol Sci* **216**, 153-162.

Jensen, I. (1975). Temporal lobe epilepsy. Late mortality in patients treated with unilateral temporal lobe resections. *Acta Neurol Scand* **52**, 374-380.

Johnston, S.C., Horn, J.K., Valente, J. and Simon, R.P. (1995). The role of hypoventilation in a sheep model of epileptic sudden death. *Ann Neurol* **37**, 531-537.

Johnston, S.C., Siedenberg, R., Min, J.K., Jerome, E.H. and Laxer, K.D. (1997). Central apnea and acute cardiac ischemia in a sheep model of epileptic sudden death. *Ann Neurol* **42**, S88-04.

Kennebäck, G., Ericson, M., Tomson, T. and Bergfeldt, L. (1997). Changes in arrhythmia profile and heart rate variability during abrupt withdrawal of antiepileptic drugs. Implications for sudden death. *Seizure* **6**, 369-375.

Kloster, R. and Engelskjon, T. (1999). Sudden unexpected death in epilepsy: a clinical perspective and a search for risk factors. *J Neurol Neurosurg Psychiatry* **67**, 439-444.

Langan, Y., Nashef, L. and Sander, J.W.A.S. (2000). Sudden unexpected death in epilepsy: a series of witnessed deaths. *J Neurol Neurosurg Psychiatry* **68**, 211-213.

Langan, Y., Nashef, L. and Sander, J.W. (2005). Case-control study of SUDEP. *Neurology* **64**, 1131-1133.

Leestma, J.E., Walczak, T., Hughes, J.R., Kalelkar, M.B. and Teas, S.S. (1989). A prospective study on sudden unexpected death in epilepsy. *Ann Neurol* **26**, 195-203.

Lhatoo, S.D., Johnson, A.L., Goodridge, D.M., MacDonald, B.K., Sander, J.W. and Shorvon, S.D. (2001). Mortality in epilepsy in the first 11 to 14 years after diagnosis: multivariate analysis of a long-term, prospective, population-based cohort. *Ann Neurol* **49**, 336-344.

Lund, A. and Gormsen, H. (1985). The role of anti-epileptics in sudden death in epilepsy. *Acta Neurol Scand* **72**, 444-446.

Massetani, R., Strata, G., Galli, R. *et al.* (1997). Alteration of cardiac function in patients with temporal lobe epilepsy: different roles of EEG-ECG monitoring and spectral analysis of RR variability. *Epilepsia* **38**, 363-369.

Morton, B., Richardson, A. and Duncan, S. (2006). Sudden unexpected death in epilepsy (SUDEP): don't ask, don't tell. *J Neurol Neurosurg Psychiatry* **77**, 199-202.

(MRC) Medical Research Council. (1991). Antiepileptic Drug Withdrawal Study Group Randomized study of antiepileptic drug withdrawal in patients in remission. *Lancet* **337**, 1175-1180.

Nashef, L., (1997). Sudden Unexpected Death in Epilepsy: Terminology and Definitions. *Epilepsia* **38 (Suppl 11)**, S6-S8.

Nashef, L. (2004). Sudden death in Epilepsy. In: Fish, D., Dodson, E. , Perucca, E. and Shorvon S. (Eds), *The Treatment of Epilepsy* . (2nd edition). Blackwell Science. pp43-49.,

Nashef, L., Fish, D.R., Garner, S., Sander, J.W.A.S. and Shorvon, S.D. (1995). Sudden Death in Epilepsy - A Study of Incidence in a Young Cohort with Epilepsy and Learning Difficulty. *Epilepsia* **36**, 1187-1194.

Nashef, L., Garner, S., Sander, J.W.A.S., Fish, D.R. and Shorvon, S.D. (1998). Circumstances of death in sudden death in epilepsy: Interviews of Bereaved Relatives. *J Neurol Neurosurg Psychiatry* **64**, 349-352.

Natelson, B.H., Suarez, R.V., Terrence, C.F. and Turizo, R. (1998). Patients with epilepsy who die suddenly have cardiac disease. *Arch Neurol* **55**, 857-860.

National Sentinel Audit of Epilepsy-Related Death. (2002). National Institute for Clinical Excellence. (www.nice.org.uk) May 2002. ISBN: 1-84257-173-7.

Nilsson, L., Farahmand, B. Y., Persson, P-G., Thiblin, I. and Tomson, T. (1999). Risk factors for sudden unexpected death in epilepsy: a case-control study. *Lancet* **353**, 888-893.

Nilsson, L., Bergman, U., Diwan, V., Farahmand, B.Y., Persson, P.G. and Tomson, T. (2001). Antiepileptic drug therapy and its management in sudden unexpected death in epilepsy: a case-control study. *Epilepsia* **42**, 667-673.

Nilsson, L., Ahl bom, A., Farahmand, B.Y. and Tomson, T. (2003). Mortality in a population-based cohort of epilepsy surgery patients. *Epilepsia* **44**, 575-581.

O'Donoghue, M.F. and Sander, J.W.A.S. (1997). The mortality associated with epilepsy, with particular reference to sudden unexpected death: a review. *Epilepsia* **38(Suppl 11)**, S15-S19.

Opeskin, K., Burke, M.P., Cordner, S.M. and Berkovic, S.F. (1999). Comparison of antiepileptic drug levels in sudden unexpected deaths in epilepsy with deaths from other causes. *Epilepsia* **40**, 1795-1798.

Opeskin, K., Thomas, A. and Berkovic, S.F. (2000). Does cardiac conduction pathology contribute to sudden unexpected death in epilepsy? *Epilepsy Res* **40**, 17-24.

Persson, H., Ericson, M. and Tomson, T. (2003). Carbamazepine affects autonomic cardiac control in patients with newly diagnosed epilepsy. *Epilepsy Res* **57**, 69-75.

Persson, H., Kumlien, E., Ericson, M. and Tomson, T. (2005). Preoperative heart rate variability in relation to surgery outcome in refractory epilepsy. *Neurology* **65**, 1021-1025.

Pomeranz, B., Macaulay, R.J., Caudill, M.A. *et al.* (1985). Assessment of autonomic function in humans by heart rate spectral analysis. *Am J Physiol* **248**, H151-153.

Rocamora, R., Kurthen, M., Lickfett, L., Von Oertzen, J. and Elger, C.E. (2003). Cardiac asystole in epilepsy: clinical and neurophysiologic features. *Epilepsia* **44**, 179-185.

Ronkainen, E., Ansakorpi, H., Huikuri, H.V., Myllylä, V.V., Isojärvi, J.I.T. and Korpelainen, J.T. (2005). Suppressed circadian heart rate dynamics in temporal lobe epilepsy. *J Neurol Neurosurg Psychiatry* **76**, 1382-1386.

Rugg-Gunn, F.J., Simister, R.J., Squirrell, M., Holdright, D.R. and Duncan, J.S. (2004). Cardiac arrhythmias in focal epilepsy: a prospective long-term study. *Lancet*. **364**, 2212-2219.

Ryvlin, P. and Kahane, P. (2003). Does epilepsy surgery lower the mortality of drug-resistant epilepsy? *Epilepsy Res* **56**, 105-120.

Salanova, V., Markand, O. and Worth, R. (2002). Temporal lobe epilepsy surgery: outcome, complications, and late mortality rate in 215 patients. *Epilepsia* **43**, 170-174.

Sillanpää, M., Jalava, M., Kaleva, O. and Shinnar, S. (1998). Long-term prognosis of seizures with onset in childhood. *N Engl J Med.* **338**, 1715-1722.

Sperling, M.R., Feldman, H., Kinman, J. *et al.* (1999). Seizure control and mortality in epilepsy. *Ann Neurol* **46**, 45-50.

Sperling, M.R., Harris, A., Nei, M., Liporice, J.D. and O'Connor, M.J. (2005). Mortality after epilepsy surgery. *Epilepsia* **46(Suppl 11)**, 49-53.

Stavem, K. and Guldvog, B. (2005). Long-term survival after epilepsy surgery compared with matched epilepsy controls and the general population. *Epilepsy Res* **63**, 67-75.

Stollberger, C. and Finsterer, J. (2004). Cardiorespiratory findings in sudden unexplained/unexpected death in epilepsy (SUDEP). *Epilepsy Res* **59**, 51-60.

Takase, B., Kurita, A., Noritake, M. *et al.* (1992). Heart rate variability in patients with diabetes mellitus, ischemic heart disease, and congestive heart failure. *J Electrocardiol* **25**, 79-88.

Taylor, D.C. and Marsh, S.M. (1977). Implications of long-term follow-up studies in epilepsy: with a note on the cause of death. In: Penry, J. K. (Ed), *Epilepsy, the Eighth International Symposium.* Raven Press, New York. pp27-34.

Thom, M. (1997). Neuropathologic findings in postmortem studies of sudden death in epilepsy *Epilepsia* **38(Suppl 11)**, S32-S34.

Timmings, P.L. (1998). Sudden unexpected death in epilepsy: is carbamazepine implicated? *Seizure* **7**, 289-291.

Tomson, T., Ericson, M., Ihrman, C. *et al.* (1998). Heart rate variability in patients with epilepsy. *Epilepsy Res* **30**, 77-83.

Tomson, T., Skold, A.C., Holmgen, P., Nilsson, L. and Danielsson, B. (1998). Postmortem changes in blood concentrations of phenytoin and carbamazepine: an experimental study. *Ther Drug Monit* **20**, 309-312.

Tomson, T., Walczak, T., Sillanpää, M. and Sander, J.W.A.S. (2005). Sudden unexpected death in epilepsy: A review of incidence and risk factors. *Epilepsia* **46(Suppl 11)**, S54-61.

Ulrich, J. and Maxeiner, H. (2003). Tongue bite injuries—a diagnostic criterium for death in epileptic seizure? *Arch Kriminol* **212**, 19-29. (English abstract; Article in German).

Vickrey, B.G. (1997). Mortality in a consecutive cohort of 248 adolescents and adults who underwent diagnostic evaluation for epilepsy surgery. *Epilepsia* **38 (Suppl 11)**, S67.

Vickrey, B.G., Hays, R.D., Rausch, R., Engel, J., Visscher, B.R., Ary, C.M., Rogers, W.H. and Brook, R.H. (1995). Outcomes in 248 patients who had diagnostic evaluations for epilepsy surgery. *Lancet* **346**, 1445-1449.

Walczak, T. (2003). Do antiepileptic drugs play a role in sudden unexpected death in epilepsy? *Drug Saf* **26**, 673-683.

Walczak, T.S., Leppik, I.E., D'Amelio, M., Rarick, J., So, E., Ahman, P., Ruggles, K., Cascino, G.D., Annegers, J.F. and Hauser, W.A. (2001). Incidence & risk factors in sudden unexpected death in epilepsy: a prospective cohort study. *Neurology* **56**, 519-525.

Weber, P., Bubl, R., Blauenstein, U., Tillmann, B.U. and Lutschg, J. (2005). Sudden unexplained death in children with epilepsy: A cohort study with an eighteen-year follow-up. *Acta Paediatr* **94**, 564-567.

Williams, J., Lawthom, C., Dunstan, F.D., Dawson, T.P., Kerr, M.P., Wilson, J.F. and Smith, P.E. (2006). Variability of antiepileptic medication taking behaviour in sudden unexplained death in epilepsy: hair analysis at autopsy. *J Neurol Neurosurg Psychiatry* **77**, 481-484.

Yang, T.S., Wong, T.T., Chang, K.P., Kwan, S.Y., Kuo, W.Y., Lee, Y.C. and Kuo, T.B.J. (2001). Power spectrum analysis of heart rate variability in children with epilepsy. *Child's Nerv Syst* **17**, 602-606.

Seizure Freedom: Clinical, Research and Quality of Life Perspectives
Edited by Michael R. Trimble
© 2006 Clarius Press Ltd

8

Treatment Resistance
in Epilepsy

PETER KINIRONS and NORMAN DELANTY

Department of Clinical Neurological Science
Royal College of Surgeons of Ireland,
Beaumont Hospital,
Dublin, Ireland

INTRODUCTION

Although no single accepted definition of pharmacoresistant epilepsy exists, most experts would agree that, broadly speaking, it is epilepsy in which seizures are not fully controlled for at least 12-month period by the use of maximally tolerated doses of currently available anticonvulsant medications, either alone or in combination (Perucca, 1998). Some authors would go further and say that if patients fail to respond to two appropriate anti-epileptic drugs (AEDs), then they are drug-resistant. This is based on evidence that suggests that the likelihood of responding to another AED, having failed two, is less than 10%. (Brodie, 2004). However, as new AEDs with novel target sites become available, this thinking may have to be revised.

It is important to recognise that not being seizure-free is not always equiv-alent to drug-resistance, as there are many other potential causes of the former, including inappropriate dosing and compliance. Currently it is estimated that between 20 and 40% of patients with epilepsy are resistant to AEDs (Kwan *et al.*, 2000; Annegers *et al.*, 1979; Forsgren *et al.*, 1995; Cockerell *et al.*, 1995). As epilepsy affects approximately 1% of the population, it is clear that this represents a major public health problem, both in terms of resources on the health system and in terms of patient mortality, which is estimated to be 4-7 times higher in drug-resistant epilepsy. (Sperling *et al.*, 2004). Although a number of risk factors for drug-resistance have been identified, it is currently unclear why some patients are resistant to AEDs while others, with seemingly identical clinical syndromes, respond well to medication. This chapter will give an overview of these recognised clinical risk factors; discuss the currently hypothesised neurobiological mechanisms of pharmacoresistance; and suggest treatment strategies available for the management of this challenging condition.

EPIDEMIOLOGY OF DRUG RESISTANCE

The exact prevalence of drug-resistant epilepsy has been difficult to quantify as studies vary in their design (prospective versus retrospective), their study population (adults versus children) and their case ascertainment (hospital versus community-based). The definition of drug-resistance in these studies can also vary. However, as mentioned above, the prevalence of drug-resistance is generally estimated at about 30% of patients with epilepsy.

Until the introduction of modern AEDs, which began with phenobarbital, the ability to control seizures had been regarded with even more pessimism. Hippocrates believed that seizures beginning in adulthood lasted until death, while Gowers conceded that the spontaneous cessation of seizures is 'an event too rare to be anticipated in any given case'. The advent of medical and surgical treatment options for patients with epilepsy has clearly impacted on prognosis, and recent prospective long term outcome studies suggest a somewhat more favourable picture. The National General Practice Study of Epilepsy, a prospective population-based study of 1091 patients attending GPs with definite or possible epilepsy (Cockerell *et al.*, 1997), reported that 68% of definite cases achieved three-year remission while 54% achieved five-year remission. A prospective hospital-based study of 525 adult patients from Scotland estimated that the majority of patients became seizure-free, while 37% of their cohort was drug-resistant (Kwan *et al.*, 2000). In a population-based study of 176 children from Finland, 64% were in remission after long-term follow-up (Sillanpää *et al.*, 1999). What is clear from these studies is that some subtypes of epilepsy are more likely to be drug-resistant and that within these different subtypes, particular clinical features are associated with a greater risk of drug-resistance.

CLINICAL FEATURES ASSOCIATED WITH
GREATER RISK OF PHARMACORESISTANCE

In general, symptomatic generalised epilepsy is more likely to be drug-resistant than symptomatic focal epilepsy, which in turn has a worse prognosis than idiopathic generalised epilepsy (Kwan *et al.*, 2000; Annegers *et al.*, 1979; Forsgren *et al.*, 1995; Cockerell *et al.*, 1995, Sillanpää *et al.*, 1999; Regesta *et al.*,

1999; Semah *et al.*, 1999). Sillanpää's long-term follow up of 176 children found that 78% of symptomatic generalised epilepsy was drug resistant, compared to 49% of symptomatic focal epilepsy and 13% of idiopathic generalised epilepsy (Sillanpää *et al.*, 1999). In their study, Kwan and Brodie classified epilepsy somewhat differently, and found that 43% of patients with symptomatic epilepsy with a known cause were drug resistant versus 39% of 'cryptogenic' (presumed symptomatic though cause unknown) cases and 26% of idiopathic cases (Kwan *et al.*, 2000). A further follow-up study from this group looking at focal epilepsy where the cause was known, found that patients with mesial temporal sclerosis were more likely to be drug resistant (58%) than patients with cortical dysplasia (46%), cerebral atrophy (45%), cortical gliosis (43%), primary brain tumour (37%), cerebral infarction (33%), or arteriovenous malformations (22%) (Kwan *et al.*, 2001).

Despite this, there is, as yet, no clear evidence to suggest that the presence of hippocampal sclerosis is more likely to be associated with drug-resistance in patients with mesial temporal lobe epilepsy (Kim *et al.*, 1999; Kumlien *et al.*, 2002; Andrade-Valenca *et al.*, 2003). Several studies, mainly from tertiary referral centres and surgical series, closely linked drug-resistance to the presence of hippocampal sclerosis (Van Paesschen *et al.*, 1997; Lehericy *et al.*, 1997). However, such interpretation may have been biased because of a higher prevalence of more severe cases at these centres and because patients with good seizure control may not undergo sophisticated neuroimaging. Some reports have shown the presence of hippocampal sclerosis in those with good seizure control (Kim *et al.*, 1999; Kumlien *et al.*, 2002; Andrade-Valenca *et al.*, 2003). As more patients undergo more advanced neuroimaging; picking up more subtle cases, a clearer picture of the prognosis associated with hippocampal sclerosis should emerge.

Other risk factors for drug-resistance that have been identified by some authors include earlier onset of seizures (Annegers *et al.*, 1979; Sofijanov *et al.*, 1982); greater number of seizures prior to treatment; high frequency of seizures from onset (Sillanpää *et al.*, 1993; Camfield *et al.*, 1994); multiple seizure types (Hauser *et al.*, 1992) history of status epilepticus (Sillanpää *et al.*, 1993); presence of neurological impairment (Aicardi *et al.*, 1990); and the presence of gross EEG abnormalities (Rowan *et al.*, 1980).

Along with these recognised risk factors, a number of patterns of drug-resistance have been observed clinically and these have suggested different theories for the development of drug-resistance (Shorvon *et al.*, 1986; Kwan *et al.*, 2001; Berg *et al.*, 2003). The 'de novo' theory claims that drug-resistance is developed before any AEDs are administered and is a feature of the epilepsy syndrome from the onset. This theory is based on observations that most drug-resistant patients fail to respond to their very first AED (Kwan *et al.*, 2000; Camfield *et al.*, 1997; Brodie *et al.*, 2004). In fact it has been shown that only 7% of patients who fail to respond to their first two AEDs achieve remission, and this decreases to 3% for patients who have failed three AEDs (Brodie, 2004). Thus these patients tend to be resistant to most, if not all, AEDs. This is important, considering many of these drugs have different mechanisms of action and implies that there is something abnormal about the underlying epileptic tissue (see later).

Most drug resistant patients appear to fall into this category. However, some patients appear to develop drug-resistance several years after their initial seizures were easily controlled (Berg et al., 2003; Brodie et al., 2004). Brodie and colleagues reported that, overall, 9% of initially responsive patients went on to become pharmacoresistant (Brodie, 2004) while a study in children found a similar outcome in 4% (Berg et al., 2003). This is particularly noticeable in patients with mesial temporal lobe epilepsy. A not unfamiliar pattern with this type of epilepsy is for patients to develop seizures in child-hood or early teens that are very responsive to medication, sometimes even allowing drug withdrawal, only for drug-resistant seizures to recur after a variable latent period. This has been referred to as the 'stuttering' course of mesial TLE (Engel, 1987). These observations suggest that mesial TLE may be a progressive disorder, at least in some patients. The initial seizures may act as an insult, which then causes morphologic and functional changes resulting in the development of drug-resistant epileptic neuronal circuits. There is both animal and neuroimaging data to support this hypothesis (Sutula et al., 2003; Briellmann et al., 2002; Fuerst et al., 2003).

The third clinically observed pattern is in patients who initially appear to be drug-resistant but then go into remission, albeit transiently in some cases (Shorvon et al., 1986). In many patients this may be due to the addition of a new, modern AED, seen most clearly in clinical trials of levetiracetam and pregabalin as add-on therapy in partial epilepsy, where remission rates of 8% and 5% were seen respectively (Shorvon et al., 2000; French et al., 2003). Levetiracetam has a unique mechanism of action, acting on the synaptic vesicle protein SV2a (Lynch et al., 2004), and its benefit in a proportion of previously refractory patients may suggest something about the underlying mechanism of seizures in patients who respond. Adding new AEDs does not account for all cases who remit, however and there is a sense that in some patients, their epilepsy 'burns itself out'.

BIOLOGICAL HYPOTHESIS OF PHARMACORESISTANCE

The basis of resistance to currently available AEDs is most likely a complex, multifactorial process, with contributions from both acquired and genetic factors. While the nature of the underlying syndrome and cause undoubtedly play a role, as discussed above, these clearly do not account for the whole picture. Patients with seemingly clinically similar epilepsy types may have dramatically different responses to AEDs. Therefore, differences at the molecular level would appear to also play a role. Most current research has focused on two major hypotheses (Schmidt and Löscher, 2005). The first is that drug-resistance results from intrinsic or acquired changes in the targets for AEDs in the brain. The second is that over-expression of multi-drug efflux transporters at the blood-brain barrier or epileptic focus results in decreased availability of AEDs at their target sites. We will examine these hypotheses in further detail in the following section.

Alterations in drug targets

Although the specific aetiological cause is unknown in most forms of epilepsy, seizures result from the spontaneous, synchronous discharge of neurones. AEDs are currently developed in an attempt to control this process and therefore generally act by limiting depolarisation – either by modulating ion channels, specifically sodium or calcium channels; by enhancing the effect of the inhibitory neurotransmitter GABA; or by blocking or attenuating the effect of the excitatory neurotransmitter glutamate. Many AEDs have combinations of these actions and probably other unrecognised actions, accounting for their different clinical efficacies. Novel targets are increasingly being recognised, such as that described above for levetiracetam. The target hypothesis claims that resistance to AEDs results from alterations in these targets, reducing the effect of the drug so that it cannot prevent initiation or propagation of the seizure. These alterations are thought to result from the changes in brain molecular structure and function that occurs during the process of epileptogenesis, and that for some reason, possibly genetic, patients who are drug-resistant are more susceptible to these molecular changes in drug targets than those who are drug-sensitive.

Evidence to support this hypothesis comes from both animal and human studies. Carbamazepine (CBZ) has been shown to produce only 50% modulation of sodium current inactivation in hippocampal neurones from patients with mesial temporal sclerosis compared to both neocortical neurones from the same patient and hippocampal neurones from patients without mesial temporal sclerosis (Vreugdenhil et al., 1998). Similar findings have been observed in kindled rats compared to control rats (Vreugdenhil et al., 1999). Remy et al have shown that use-dependent blockade of voltage-dependent sodium channels, the principal mode of action of CBZ, is completely lost in carbamazepine-resistant patients compared to carbamazepine-responsive patients with TLE (Remy et al., 2003). The same group have also shown that the effects on sodium channels of phenytoin and, to a lesser extent, lamotrigine, were reduced in epileptic compared with control animals, in the rat pilocarpine model of TLE (Remy et al., 2003). These data suggest that a loss of sodium channel drug sensitivity may constitute one mechanism underlying the development of drug-resistant epilepsy. To further investigate this, Ellerkmann and colleagues (2003) looked at the expression of subunits of the sodium channel receptor in rat hippocampus after an episode of status epilepticus (S.E) and found persistent down-regulation of the pore-forming Na(v)1.2 and Na(v)1.6 subunit as well as the accessory beta(1) subunit up to 30 days following S.E. Co-expression of beta subunits is known to shift the voltage-dependence of inactivation in a hyperpolarizing direction (Isom *et al.*, 2002). Therefore down-regulation of beta-subunit expression may contribute to the depolarizing shift in the inactivation curve noted following S.E. These subunits also modulate channel gating and regulate the level of expression at the plasma membrane (Isom *et al.*, 2002). This may explain, on a molecular level, the mechanism by which AEDs that act on sodium channels are rendered ineffective.

Another common mechanism of action for AEDs is enhancement of the inhibitory GABA system. This is done in a number of different ways by different compounds – drugs such as benzodiazepines and phenbarbitone act directly on GABA receptors; vigabatrin prevents breakdown of GABA by inhibiting GABA transaminase while tiagabine blocks re-uptake of GABA by inhibiting the GABA transporter GAT 1. Other drugs such as valproate and topiramate are also thought to achieve some of their anti-convulsant properties by enhancing GABA transmission. The principal GABA receptors in the brain are $GABA_A$ receptors, which mediate fast synaptic inhibition. These are composed of pentameric ligand gated chloride channels. Although there are eight different subunit types and multiple subclasses of each subunit, by far the commonest receptor stoichiometry is $alpha_1$, $beta_2$, $gamma_2$ (Sieghart *et al.*, 2002). However many other combinations have been shown to exist and many more are theoretically possible.

These receptor subtypes display different properties in response to both GABA and exogenous compounds such as diazepam and zolpidem (Sieghart *et al.*, 2002). For example, subunits containing an alpha4 or alpha6 subunit are insensitive to benzodiazepines (Rudolph *et al.*, 2004). Therefore alterations in the subunit composition of GABA receptors may result in profound alterations in receptor function and pharmacology.

There is some evidence that these changes may contribute to drug-resistance. Many studies have shown major alterations in subunit expression both in human and animal models of TLE (Brooks-Kayal *et al.*, 1998; Sperk *et al.*, 1998; Fritschy *et al.*, 1998; Bouilleret *et al.*, 2000; Redecker *et al.*, 2000; Loup *et al.*, 2000). A recent study investigated changes in the expression of major $GABA_A$ receptor subunits ($alpha_1$, $alpha_2$, $alpha_4$, $alpha_5$, $beta_1$, $beta_3$, $gamma_2$ and delta) and of the $GABA_B$ receptor species $GABA_BR1a$, $GABA_BR1b$ and $GABA_BR2$ in 1) hippocampal kindling and 2) epilepsy following electrically-induced S.E (Nishimura *et al.*, 2005). The most prominent changes were a relatively fast and lasting reduction of delta subunit mRNA levels in dentate granule cells, accompanied by increases in mRNA levels of all three beta-subunits and subunit $gamma_2$. Levels of subunit $alpha_4$ were increased by up to 60% in dentate granule cells in both animal models, whereas those of subunit $alpha_5$ were decreased after SE, but not after kindling. In cornu ammonis 3 pyramidal cells, down-regulation of subunits $alpha_2$, $alpha_4$, $alpha_5$, and $beta_{1-3}$ was observed in the ventral hippocampus and of $alpha_2$, $alpha_5$, $beta_3$ and $gamma_2$ in its dorsal extension 24 hours after S.E. While persistent decreases in subunit $alpha_2$, $alpha_4$ and $beta_2$ transcript levels were presumably related to SE-induced cell loss, the observed changes suggest substantial and cell specific rearrangement of GABA receptors.

Another study looking at the expression of $GABA_A$ receptor subunits in seizure-prone and seizure-resistant strains of rat after status epilepticus found that $alpha_1$ subunit expression is reduced in seizure-prone rats and increased in seizure-resistant rats, thus exhibiting opposing molecular responses (Gilby *et al.*, 2005). Furthermore, rapid development of resistance to drugs that act on the $GABA_A$ receptor has been shown to occur in the rat model of pilocarpine-induced status epilepticus (Jones *et al.*, 2002). In hippocampal specimens obtained at surgery from TLE patients with and without hippocampal sclerosis, investigation of the expression of $GABA_A$ receptor subunits $alpha_1$, $alpha_3$, $beta_{1-3}$, and $gamma_2$ revealed significant decreases in all these subunits immunoreactivity in sclerotic but not in non-sclerotic specimens, consistent with the severe neurodegeneration in the CA1 sector (Pirker *et al.*, 2003). In contrast, pronounced increases in immunoreactivity of all 3 beta-subunits were observed in most sectors of the hippocampal formation both in sclerotic and nonsclerotic specimens, again indicating pronounced adaptive changes in the expression of these $GABA_A$ receptor subunits related to seizure activity.

It is clear then that changes in the composition of receptors do occur in response to seizures, at least in TLE patients. Therefore it would seem a reasonable hypothesis to propose that these changes result in decreased affinity of the target receptor for the drug or endogenous ligand. The big question, and the one that remains to be answered conclusively, is do these changes occur only, or at least to a much greater extent, in patients who are drug resistant? This remains difficult to prove. One reason for this is the obvious problem of obtaining comparative brain tissue from patients who respond to AEDs as these patients do not undergo resective surgery. Thus studies comparing the sensitivities of brain tissue to various drugs from resistant and responsive patients are very difficult to undertake. What little data there is available is somewhat conflicting and argues against alterations of drug target proteins being the sole reason for drug-resistance. For example, a study looking at the effect of valproic acid (VPA) on the transient sodium current in temporal lobe resection specimens found no difference between sclerotic and non-sclerotic tissue and concluded that drug-resistance is not associated with modulation of the sodium current by VPA (Vreugdenhil *et al.*, 1998). On the other hand, seizure activity elicited in human hippocampal slices from drug-resistant patients is insensitive to carbamazepine while, in marked contrast, the drug caused use-dependent block of sodium channels and blocked seizure activity in patients clinically responsive to it (Remy *et al.*, 2003). If this hypothesis were borne out, one potentially exciting development might be the possibility of developing new AEDs that act specifically on these altered targets (Löscher and Schmidt, 2004).

Drug transporter hypothesis

Although the target hypothesis could explain why patients do not respond to AEDs acting on certain receptors, the fact that most patients are resistant to a broad range of AEDs acting via different mechanisms has led researchers to consider the possibility that a non-specific mechanism resulting in decreased penetration of drugs into the brain might play a role. It was already known from cancer research that chemotherapy-resistant tumour cells can over-express a number of 'broad-spectrum' efflux drug transporters resulting in increased amounts of drug being expelled from the cell and hence pharma-coresistance to a range of different compounds (Gottesman *et al.*, 2002). Huge interest has now focused on the role of these transporters in drug-resistant epilepsy.

The prototype of these efflux transporters is P-glycoprotein (P-gp). This belongs to a highly conserved protein super-family, the adenosine triphos-phate-binding cassette (ABC) proteins, which has more than 100 members and is found in a wide variety of organisms (Van Veen *et al.*, 1997). These proteins function as active pumps at the cell membrane through hydrolysis of ATP to drive the flux of their substrates against the concentration gradient. They have a wide range of substrates including drugs, nutrients, amino acids, sugars, peptides, pigments and metals (Klein *et al.*, 1999). Mutations in some of these proteins can cause genetic disease in humans, such as in the trans-membrane conductance regulator (CFTR) in cystic fibrosis (Dean *et al.*, 2000).

P-gp in humans is encoded by two genes, MDR1 and MDR2, located on chromosome 7 (Callen *et al.*, 1987). MRD1 encodes the drug-transporter associated with multi-drug resistance whereas MDR2 encodes a phosphatidylcholine transporter in biliary canaliculi (Silverman *et al.*, 1999). MDR1 P-gp is an integral membrane protein comprising two homologous halves, each consisting of one transmembrane domain containing six segments and one nucleotide binding domain (Gottesman *et al.*, 2002; Dicato *et al.*, 1997). P-gp has a wide variety of known drug substrates, including anthracyclines, alkaloids, peptides, steroid hormones and local anaesthetics,

Table 1.   Examples of known drug substrates for P-glycoprotein

Anticancer Drugs	*Steroids*	*Peptides*	*Others*
Actinomycin D	Aldosterone	Gramicidin D	Digoxin
Daunorubicin	Dexamethasone	Leupeptin	Protease inhibitors
Docetaxel		Nonacin	Loperamide
Doxorubicin	*Cytotoxins*	Pepstatin A	Rhodamine 123
Etoposide	Colchicine		Triton X-100
Mitoxanthrone	Emetine		
Pacitaxel	Puromycin	*Anticonvulsants*	
Teniposide		*See table 2*	
Vinblastine			
Vincristine			

examples of which are shown in Table 1. (Sharom *et al.*, 1997; Rodríguez *et al.*, 1999; Seelig *et al.*, 1998). It remains unclear how P-gp recognises such chemically diverse compounds but substrates are typically large (molecular weight >400), hydrophobic, amphipathic, have a planar ring system and a weakly positive charge (Sharom *et al.*, 1997). In the brain, P-gp is expressed on the apical side of the choroid plexus epithelia, contributing to the blood-CSF barrier and also to the blood-brain barrier (BBB) (Rao *et al.*, 1999). Controversy exists regarding the precise subcellular location of P-gp in the capillary endothelial cells at the BBB. Theoretically its function in reducing brain uptake of drugs can be ascribed only to transporters facing the luminal side of the brain microvasculature. However, although the majority of reports do localise it to this location (Bendayan *et al.*, 2002; Demeule *et al.*, 2002; Pardridge *et al.*, 1997; Lee *et al.*, 2001), other reports have localised it to astrocytic foot processes on the anti-luminal side of the BBB (Pardridge *et al.*, 1997; Golden *et al.*, 1999). It was thought that P-gp was not normally expressed in brain parenchyma but recent *in vitro* studies suggest it may be expressed in astrocytes and microglia (Bendayan *et al.*, 2002; Ballerini *et al.*, 2002). It also appears to be expressed in disease states such as astrocytomas, TB meningitis, encephalitis and epileptogenic brain tissue (Matsumoto *et al.*, 1991; Dietzmann *et al.*, 1994; Tishler *et al.*, 1995; Aronica *et al.*, 2004; Sisodiya *et al.*, 1999; Lardizabal *et al.*, 2003; Sisodiya *et al.*, 2002; Aronica *et al.*, 2003; Lardizabal *et al.*, 2003 ; Volk *et al.*, 2004a; 2004b).

Tishler *et al* first reported over-expression of P-gp in drug-resistant epilepsy in 1995 in tissue from patients undergoing resective surgery (Tishler *et al.*, 1995). They examined MDR1 mRNA levels in 19 patients, 15 of whom had undergone temporal lobectomy, with a variety of pathologies (mostly hippocampal sclerosis). In 11 of the 19, they found levels were over ten times greater than in samples resected from patients undergoing surgery for arteriovenous malformations. They also detected P-gp in astrocytes, suggesting novel expression sites. Since then a number of reports have emerged confirming these findings in resected samples and in a variety of aetiologies, including hippocampal sclerosis (Aronica et al., 2004), cortical dysplasia (Sisodiya et al., 1999), tuberous sclerosis (Lazarowski et al., 2004), dysembryoplastic neuroepithetial tumours (DNET) (Sisodiya et al., 2002), ganglioglioma (Aronica et al., 2003) and Rasmussen's encephalitis (Lardizabal et al., 2003). Interestingly, overexpression has been detected not only in endothelial cells, but also in astrocytes and even neurons in some cases. Furthermore, increased expression of these efflux transporters has been reported in BBB and brain parenchyma of rat models of TLE such as the kindling, pilocarpine and kainate models (Volk et al., 2004a; 2004b; Zhang et al., 1999; Potschka et al., 2004). Studies of resected brain tissue suggest that overexpression is limited to the abnormal epileptic focus (Sisodiya et al., 2002; D'Giano et al., 1997).

A number of other efflux transporters have also been studied in epileptic brain tissue. Principal among these are members of the multi-drug resistance associated proteins (MRPs) and more recently major vault protein (MVP). MRP 2 and MRP 5 have been shown to be overexpressed in capillary endothelial cells from human epileptic brain tissue, while MRP 1 is overexpressed in neurons and astrocytes in these patients (Sisodiya et al., 2002; Aronica et al., 2003; Dombrowski et al., 2001). Ectopic upregulation of MVP has been detected in hilar neurons in hippocampal sclerosis, dysplastic neurons in focal cortical dysplasia, and lesional neurons in DNET, in samples taken from drug-resistant epileptic patients when compared to controls (Sisodiya et al., 2003). Thus it appears that more than one efflux transporter may be upregulated in a given epileptogenic pathology. Some 20 other efflux transporters have been recognised in a number of tissues including the brain (Langmann et al., 2003; Gao et al., 2000; Taylor et al., 2002); to what extent they may contribute to drug resistance in epilepsy is as yet unknown. The role of increased expression of these efflux transporters in epileptic brain tissue is also unclear. It possibly represents a secondary defence mechanism of the BBB because of transient BBB opening during seizures and chronic dysregulation of BBB function as indicated by endothelial cell alterations, abnormal tight junctions and thickening of the basal membrane, but the precise function of these transporters remains obscure (Schmidt et al., 2005; Cornford et al., 1999).

One interesting question is whether increased expression of these efflux transporters is an inherent feature of the abnormal brain tissue or a direct response to seizures. This is important because, if the latter is the case, ongoing seizures may actually contribute to the development of drug-resistance. Clinical studies showing an increased risk of drug-resistance with a greater number of seizures prior to treatment would support this (Shorvon et *al.*, 1982; Elwes *et al.*, 1984). The presence of similar findings of overexpression across a range of pathologic lesions is also supportive, as are studies in animals showing increased expression of P-gp in response to seizures (Volk *et al.*, 2004a; 2004b; Seegers *et al.*, 2002). Although these data are far from conclusive, they may suggest that early, aggressive management of seizures is important in helping to prevent the development of drug resistance.

As in the case of the target hypothesis, one of the main obstacles to proving a role for increased expression of P-gp and other transporters in pharmacoresistance is the difficulty in obtaining comparative 'control' tissue from drug-sensitive patients. If, for example, expression of P-gp could be shown to be several times higher in drug-resistant patients with hippocampal sclerosis than those with drug-sensitive hippocampal sclerosis, this would go some way to proving this hypothesis. This appears unlikely to happen unless *in vivo* techniques can be developed.

A second difficulty in proving this hypothesis is establishing that AEDs are actual substrates for these transporters. The fact that a number of AEDs are large, hydrophobic substances makes them potential candidates. However use of different methodologies to study uptake of drugs by transporters has made interpretation of results difficult (Kwan *et al.*, 2005). For example, transporter-expressing cell lines allow high throughput screening but only with *in vitro* analysis. Co-administration of an inhibitor to determine effects on drug uptake allows *in vivo* and *in vitro* analysis but these inhibitors tend to lack specificity for individual transporters. Knockout mice are also used but problems arise because of the wide tissue distribution of P-gp (Schinkel *et al.*, 1997) and also because it is possible that compensatory mechanisms may arise that cloud the function of the transporter. For example expression of MDR1b is upregulated in MDR1a knock-outs (Schinkel *et al.*, 1994). However, there is some evidence to suggest that the following AEDs are substrates for P-gp (see Table 2): phenytoin (Potschka *et al.*, 2001; Rizzi *et al.*, 2002), carbamazepine (Potschka *et al.*, 2001; Sills *et al.*, 2002), phenobarbital (Potschka *et al.*, 2002), felbamate (Potschka *et al.*, 2002), lamotrigine (Potschka *et al.*, 2002), gabapentin (Luer *et al.*, 1999), and topiramate (Sills *et al.*, 2002), while phenytoin, carbamazepine and valproate may also be substrates for the MRPs (100,104,105). Evidence is conflicting for some of these drugs, for example carbamazepine. Three groups have independently found evidence of transport by P-gp (Potschska *et al.*, 2001; Sills *et al.*, 2002; Rizzi *et al.*, 2002) whereas one study did not (Owen *et al.*, 2001). Furthermore, levetiracetam does not appear to be a substrate for either of these transporters (Potschka *et al.*, 2004) while it is not known whether oxcarbazepine, vigabatrin, pregabalin, zonismide, tiagabine or ethosuximide are substrates for multi-drug transporters. This is further evidence against the drug transporter hypothesis as most patients who are resistant to known P-gp substrates are also resistant to levetiracetam.

Table 2.   Current evidence that AEDs are substrates for efflux drug transporters. (Y=yes, N=no, N/S=not studied)

Drug	P-gp	MRP	Ref.
Carbamazepine	Y	Y	Potschka *et al.*, 2001; Sills *et al.*, 2002
Felbamate	Y	N	Potschka *et al.*, 2002
Gabapentin	Y	N/S	Sills *et al.*, 2002
Lamotrigine	Y	N	Potschka *et al.*, 2002
Levetiracetam	N	N	Potschka *et al.*, 2004
Phenobarbitone	Y	N	Potschka *et al.*, 2002; Potschka *et al.*, 2003
Phenytoin	Y	Y	Potschka *et al.*, 2001, 2002; Rizzi et al 2002
Topiramate	Y	N/S	Sills *et al.*, 2002
Valproate	N/S	Y	Gibbs *et al.*, 2004

Thus, as with the target hypothesis, there are flaws in the transporter hypothesis. However, these findings are exciting and could potentially have important implications for our understanding of the neurobiology of epilepsy. As well as suggesting the importance of early, aggressive management of seizures, as discussed above, it is also possible that designing specific inhibitors for these transporters might allow novel treatment strategies to be devised. Indeed some early, anecdotal reports are beginning to emerge on the benefit of verapamil, a P-gp inhibitor, in the treatment of patients with drug-resistant epilepsy (Summers *et al.*, 2004; Iannetti *et al.*, 2005). Although the transporter hypothesis may not fully explain pharmacoresistance, it seems likely that it could be one of the important contributing factors.

GENETICS OF PHARMACORESISTANCE

If differences exist in the alteration of drug targets and/or the expression of drug transporters between drug-sensitive and drug-resistant patients, what factors result in this difference? It seems likely that inherent differences in the way patients respond to seizures may play a role. Thus genetic differences between responders and non-responders make for an attractive hypothesis. Genetic contributions to common conditions are typically made up of rare mutations of strong effect, which contribute a minor amount to the overall prevalence of a condition, and common genetic variants, particularly single nucleotide polymorphisms (SNP), which may be of more modest effect but in combination with each other and with environmental factors may be enough to result in a particular phenotype and are likely to contribute much more to the overall prevalence. It is this latter area that is the focus of much current research into drug resistance in epilepsy. It must be noted however that the genetics of drug resistance may differ somewhat from the genetics of disease, in which disease causing mutations will be 'selected out' over time, resulting in their very low frequency in the population. Mutations affecting drug transport proteins, for example, may not be under such negative selection pressures as they may have been 'clinically silent' before the use of current drugs or may even be under positive selection pressures if they have a role in protecting the brain from toxins.

A small number of mutations have been found to associate with drug-resistance. Mutations in the sodium channel genes, SCN1A and SCN1B, have been found not only to result in epilepsy, but also epilepsy that is resistant to drug treatment (Ceulemans *et al.*, 2004; Kamiya *et al.*, 2004). Although functional studies confirming the mechanism of the altered subunit's diminished response to AEDs are lacking, the fact that many AEDs exert their effects primarily through their action on sodium channels makes this a biologically plausible result. This evidence provides further support to the target hypothesis. As yet, evidence to support a role for common variation in the sodium channel genes and drug-resistance is lacking. A recent study looking at variants in the genes for the subunits SCN1A, SCN2A, SCN3A, SCN8A, SCN1B, SCN2B, in over 400 patients did not find an association between any SNPs in these genes and drug-resistance although a weak association was found for haplotypes generated for SCN3A (Depondt *et al.*, 2005).

Table 3.   Summary of studies of refractory epilepsy and ABCB1 / MDR Protein genotype
(R = responder; NR = non-responder; SZ = seizure)

Authors	*Responder (n)*	*Non-Responder (n)*	*Definition*	*Result*
Siddiqui *et al* 2003	115	200	R: Sz free > 1 yr NR: > 4 szs in last yr	Positive
Zimprich *et al* 2004	0	210	NR: 'A' < 2 szs/mth; 'B' > 2 and < 6 szs/mth; 'C' > 6 szs/mth	Positive
Tan *et al* 2004	208	401	As Siddiqui *et al*	Negative
Sills *et al* 2005	170	230	R: Sz free > 1 yr NR: All with any szs	Negative
Hung *et al* 2005	223	108	R: Sz free > 2 yrs NR: > 10 szs / year	Positive
Shahwan *et al* (Unpub)	242	198	R: Sz free or > 50% reduction in last year NR: < 50% reduction	Negative

To date mutations in multi-drug transporter proteins have not been identified. However, a lot of interest has focused on the role of common genetic variants in these genes in predisposing to drug resistant epilepsy. Most of this has stemmed from an original report of an association of a SNP in the gene for P-gp (MDR1) and drug resistant epilepsy (Siddiqui *et al.*, 2003). Since then however there have been a number of studies published which have been unable to replicate this finding (see Table 3). Thus, although this represents an attractive biologic hypothesis, the initial result may represent a false positive finding and illustrates the importance of replication before drawing conclusions on these associations. It must be noted, however, that there were some differences in the definitions of drug-resistance in these studies that may have confounded the results due to differences in the phenotype under study. Similarly, only certain AEDs are substrates for PGP and thus more careful definition of the phenotype, including a history of drug-exposure, may help to clarify the role of variation in this gene in drug-resistance. As further studies emerge looking at the role of these and other proteins involved in the pharmacology of AEDs, as well as novel candidates suggested by genome wide screening, the importance of common genetic variation in drug-resistance should become apparent.

MANAGEMENT OF PHARMACORESISTANT EPILEPSY

Despite the advances in recent years in understanding the pathogenic nature of epilepsy, as well as the release of several AEDS with novel mechanisms of action and improvements in surgical techniques, management of patients with drug-resistance remains a difficult clinical problem. This section will outline some of the current strategies available and also outline some exciting areas of current research.

Drug therapy

As discussed above, once patients have failed to respond to two appropriate AEDs, the likelihood of responding to further AEDs appears to less than 10%. However this still leaves a group of patients who will respond to further trials of particular AED or combinations of AEDs. Both clinical experience and drug trials have shown that this response can be quite dramatic. For example pivotal trials looking at levetiracetam and pregabalin as add-on therapy in refractory patients showed that 8% and 5% of patients respectively were rendered seizure-free (Shorvon *et al.*, 2000; French *et al.*,

2003), at least over the course of the trial. Therefore perseverance with trials of new AEDs is indicated in all patients. Conversely, AEDs, which have clearly not been of benefit to the patient, should be weaned. As a general rule each drug should be slowly increased to the maximum tolerated dose with careful monitoring of seizure diaries before it is discontinued.

One interesting topic is whether some drugs have a 'synergistic' effect when used in combination, i.e. the observed effect of drug A and drug B together is greater than would be expected from the known efficacies of each individually. This also raises the issue of 'rational polytherapy' which, broadly speaking, is the use of combinations of AEDs with known, although often poorly understood, pharmacodynamic interactions, or the use of AEDs with known different mechanisms of action to attempt a 'double hit' on the patient's seizures. For example, instead of using two drugs that act predominantly by blocking sodium channels, such as carbamazepine and phenytoin, one might choose a drug that affected calcium channels, such as pregabalin, or synaptic transmission, such as levetiracetam, in addition to a sodium channel blocker. One difficulty with this is that many AEDs, e.g. topiramate or valproate, have several different mechanisms of action without apparent superior efficacy over drugs with a single mechanism of action. However, the use of newer AEDs with more specific mechanisms of action may allow true rational polytherapy in this manner.

Animal studies have provided useful evidence of positive pharmacodynamic interactions involving some AEDs and results from *in vitro* studies are also promising (Luszczki *et al.*, 2005; Cuadrado *et al.*, 2005; Sills *et al.*, 2004), although there is still little evidence of the applicability of such interactions in humans. However, anecdotal evidence and clinical experience has shown that some combinations of AEDs are more effective in controlling seizures than either drug used alone. Examples of these AED combinations include valproate (VPA) and ethosuximide (ESM); clonazepam (CZP) plus VPA; carbamazepine (CBZ) plus VPA; tiagabine (TGB) plus vigabatrin (VGB); VGB plus lamotrigine (LTG); LTG plus topiramate (TPM) and VPA plus LTG (Luszczki *et al.*, 2005). Low doses of LTG coadministered with VPA appear to produce a therapeutically desirable pharmacodynamic interaction in patients with generalised seizures. (Patsalos *et al.*, 2003). However, the possibility that some of these therapeutic enhancements result from pharmacokinetic interactions taking place in the central brain compartment, rather than as a result of pharmacodynamic interactions, cannot be ruled out. Clearly, prospective randomised controlled trials are needed to further evaluate the benefits of different combinations of AEDs.

Another exciting possibility for future pharmacological therapy, and a growing area of research, is the identification of genetic markers that are known to alter the pharmacology of a drug ('pharmacogenetics'). For example, a polymorphism in a transport molecule for a hydrophilic drug might result in impaired uptake of that drug into the CNS and hence reduced efficacy of that drug. Thus, identification of these markers in patients might allow for prediction of responders and non-responders and hence more rational and individual-based prescribing of drugs or more rapid consideration of alternative treatment strategies such as surgery.

Surgery

Resective surgery in well-selected patients currently represents the best option for patients with drug-resistant epilepsy. Long-term follow-up studies of patients undergoing epilepsy surgery have reported that between 50-80 % will be rendered seizure-free (Spencer et al., 2005; Yoon et al., 2003; Tellez-Zenteno et al., 2005; Jutila et al., 2002; McIntosh et al., 2004; Jeong et al., 2005; see also Chapter 5 – this book). Patients with a better outcome appear to be younger, have no history of secondary generalised convulsions, and have imaging evidence of unilateral hippocampal sclerosis. Patient selection and careful pre-surgical work-up to identify the seizure focus are key elements in successful outcome.

It remains unclear if and for how long patients need to stay on AEDs after surgery. Logically one might suppose that successful removal of the seizure focus would obviate the need for on-going AED treatment. However clinical experience tells us that this is not always the case and attempted withdrawal of medication may result in a recurrence of seizures. Potential causes include incomplete resection of the original focus, surgical scar tissue resulting in a new focus, and patients with multiple foci. Often the precise cause is unclear. Currently there are no clear guidelines on the timing of post-operative reduction of medication. However, many clinicians would favour an observation period of at least a year before beginning to wean medication. One serious concern is that if seizures do in fact result in increased expression of multi-drug transporters, then the recurrence of seizures in these patients may set up a vicious circle of increasing drug-resistance and hence increasing seizures, a pattern which is not infrequently observed in post-operative patients. The authors would therefore recommend early, aggressive treatment of any seizures recurring in patients after epilepsy surgery.

Vagus nerve stimulation

For patients who fail drug therapy and who are not surgical candidates, the use of vagus nerve stimulation (VNS) is an alternative approach. The first reports of the benefit of VNS as a treatment for seizures began to appear in 1990 (Penry et al., 1990). The idea to stimulate the vagus nerve and disrupt or prevent seizures was proposed by Jacob Zabarra (Terry et al., 1990). He observed a consistent finding among several animal studies that indicated that stimulation of the vagus nerve could alter the EEG patterns of the animals under study. His hypothesis formed the basis for the development of the vagus nerve stimulator, a device that is implanted in the left chest and attached to the left vagus nerve via a stimulating lead. Once implanted, the stimulator is programmed to deliver regular stimulation 24 hours a day regardless of seizure activity. Patients can also activate extra 'on-demand' stimulation with a handheld magnet. Experiments in humans began in 1988 with two single-blind pilot studies that demonstrated the feasibility and safety of this therapy (Penry *et al.*, 1990; Uthman *et al.*, 1990). Following these studies, two multicenter, active-control, parallel, double-blind protocols showed a statistically significant reduction in partial onset seizures with reasonable and well-tolerated side effects (Vagus Nerve Stimulation Study Group, 1995; Salinsky *et al.*, 1996). Since then several clinical studies have demonstrated VNS therapy to be a safe and effective mode of treatment when added to the existing regimen of severe, refractory patients with epilepsy (Amar *et al.*, 1999, Lundgren *et al.*, 1998; Handforth *et al.*, 1998; Labar *et al.*, 1998).

The device was initially indicated as an add-on treatment for seizures of partial onset with or without secondary generalisation but is increasingly being used to treat other epilepsy types. Efficacy ranges from seizure-free to no response with approximately 40-50% reporting at least a 50% improvement in number of seizures after 1.5 years of treatment. The side-effect profile includes stimulation-related sensations in the neck and throat, such as cough or hoarseness. These side effects tend to reduce with time.

The mechanism of action for VNS is not clearly understood although two theories have emerged (Ben-Menachem *et al.*, 1996). First, the direct connection theory hypothesises that the anti-seizure action of VNS is caused by a seizure threshold-raising effect of the connections of the vagus nerve to the nucleus of the solitary tract and on to other structures. The second is the concept that chronic stimulation of the vagus nerve increases the amount of inhibitory neurotransmitters and decreases the amount of excitatory neurotransmitters.

One area of debate in VNS therapy is the optimum settings for patient response. While evidence suggests that, in general, a higher stimulation paradigm is better than a low one (Privitera *et al* 2002), it is becoming apparent that individual patients respond differently to various VNS settings. A recent study comparing three different level settings, including the standard setting, found no difference in overall response (DeGiorgio *et al.*, 2005). Our own practice is to start with an 'on time' of 30 seconds and an 'off time' of 1.8 minutes and gradually increase the output current until the maximum response is achieved. If seizures continue despite increasing to the maximum tolerated current, we then begin to switch to a more rapid cycle.

Dietary treatments

Dietary therapies represent a potentially valuable adjunct to other epilepsy treatments. Although the ketogenic diet (KD - high fat, adequate protein, low carbohydrate) is the most well established dietary therapy for epilepsy, other possible approaches include the Atkins diet (high fat, high protein, low carbohydrate); a diet enriched in polyunsaturated fatty acids; or overall restriction of calorie intake.

The ketogenic diet was initially devised in 1921 to mimic the anticonvulsant effects of fasting, which were known to suppress seizures (Wilder *et al.*, 1921). It was used extensively until anticonvulsant drugs (AEDs) became available in the 1930's, then fell out of favour until its resurgence in the 1990's as a treatment for drug-resistant patients. It is still used primarily in children.

The clinical efficacy of the KD has been verified in many studies (Freeman *et al.*, 1998; Vining *et al.*, 1998; Katyal *et al.*, 2000; Coppola *et al.*, 2002). In general, at least half of all patients treated with the KD will exhibit a 50% or greater reduction of seizure frequency, suggesting it is at least as good as the "new" AEDs. Any seizure type may respond to the diet, but some generalized seizure types (e.g., myoclonic, atonic, generalized tonic–clonic, and even infantile spasms) may be reduced preferentially (Maydell *et al.*, 2001). Interestingly, recent data indicate that a KD sometimes can be discontinued without concomitant loss of seizure control suggesting that it might be both anticonvulsant and antiepileptogenic (Hemingway *et al.*, 2001). The mechanism of action of the KD remains unclear. Fat breakdown in the liver creates ketone bodies (β-hydroxybutyrate, acetoacetate, and acetone), which circulate to the brain and are taken up into cerebral tissue via specific monocarboxylate transporters. In neuronal mitochondria, ketones are metabolised to adenosine triphosphate (ATP) via the tricarboxylic acid cycle and oxidative phosphorylation. The challenge has been to understand how this energy shift results in an anticonvulsant effect. There is much current research examining this question (Yamada *et al.*, 2005; Yudkoff *et al.*, 2005; Dahlin *et al.*, 2005). The main problem with the KD is compliance as it is a difficult diet for patients to adhere to. As a result researchers have begun to look at the effect of other, less severe diets in terms of seizure control.

The Atkin's diet induces a state of ketosis by providing high fat and little carbohydrate. It is therefore theoretically possible that the Atkin's diet could enable seizure control by a mechanism similar to that of the KD. Two main differences are found between the diets. First, the Atkin's diet does not restrict calories. Second, the Atkin's diet allows large amounts of protein, which is restricted on the KD. A small case series appeared recently, supporting the effectiveness of the Atkin's diet on seizure control in six patients (Kossoff *et al.*, 2003), including three children, an adolescent and two adults. All three children and the adolescent developed ketosis,whereas neither of the two adults did. With regard to seizure control, the results were remarkable: two children and the teenager had a greater than 90% seizure reduction and remained on the diet for between four and 20 months. Significant seizure control was not achieved in one child and in either adult. Although better tolerated than the KD, issues with regard to compliance also arise with the Atkin's diet, as do concerns over its safety in the long term.

Another interesting dietary approach is a reduction in overall calorie intake. The original idea for the KD was derived from the beneficial effect that fasting had on seizures (Wilder *et al.*, 1921), and this observation has been verified more recently (Freeman *et al.*, 1999). It remains unclear whether calorie restriction can reduce the seizure burden independent of ketosis. However, recent animal studies suggest that it can (Eagles *et al.*, 2003). The cause of this effect is unclear but as with the KD probably involves complicated metabolic factors. Unfortunately, this approach is obviously impractical except for very short-term use.

The long-chain polyunsaturated fatty acids (PUFAs) of the ω-3 class (as found in certain fish oils) are necessary for the development of normal retinal and neuronal membranes, as well as for subsequent normal behaviour and cognition (Uauy *et al.*, 2001). They have been shown to exert important modulatory actions on neurons: they can decrease or increase their firing rates, alter neurotransmitter release, and modulate synaptic responses (Stafstrom, 2001). They have also been shown to reduce neuronal sodium and calcium currents and inhibit or activate potassium channels (Vreugdenhil *et al.*, 1996; Xiao *et al.*, 1999). Animal studies have shown them to have antiseizure properties. Linoleic acid, administered before kainic acid–induced seizures, protects against status epilepticus and subsequent excitotoxic hippocampal cell death (Xiao *et al.*, 1999). A mixture of PUFAs of the ω-3 and ω-6 classes was shown to raise seizure threshold in rat models (Yehuda *et al.*, 1994) while in another series of experiments using a cortical-stimulation model of seizures, long-chain PUFAs produced a transient elevation in seizure threshold, which was correlated with dynamic changes in serum PUFAs concentration (Voskuyl *et al.*, 1998).

It is thought that PUFAs may diminish seizure susceptibility by altering the lipid composition of neuronal or glial membranes, through an effect on membrane protein mobility, ionic channel function, or some metabolic mechanism (Stafstrom, 2004). Intriguingly, the KD results in higher levels of PUFAs and it has been shown that the level of at least one PUFA (arachidonic acid) correlates with improved seizure control in patients on the KD, suggesting this may be one of its mechanisms of action (Cunnane *et al.*, 2002). As of yet, however, there is little data available on the role of PUFA supplementation in patients with epilepsy. One small, unblinded study of five institutionalised patients given a daily ω-3 PUFA each morning for 6 months showed a quite dramatic seizure reduction from 1 to 14 seizures per week before the trial to 1 per month afterward (Schlanger *et al.*, 2002). While these results are obviously encouraging, there were many limitations to the study, and large well-controlled prospective studies are needed to further evaluate these substances.

Other non-pharmacological techniques

Stress and anxiety can be major provoking factors for some patients with epilepsy. The use of psychological techniques to better deal with these factors has therefore been of interest to some investigators looking for non-pharmacological ways to improve seizure control. A small number of studies have shown a significant improvement in seizure control using a range of psychological methods (Schmid-Schonbein, 1998; Muller, 2001). However a recent Cochrane review of these methods found that because of methodological deficiencies and limited number of individuals studied, there no reliable evidence to support the use of these treatments (Ramaratnam *et al.*, 2003). Other non-pharmacological techniques include various forms of biofeedback techniques. Again studies are limited and clearly further trials are needed to evaluate the role for all of these treatments.

CONCLUSIONS

Drug resistant epilepsy is a common and difficult problem, estimated to affect about one third of patients. Certain clinical features are associated with an increased risk such as the underlying cause, early onset and high frequency of seizures, and the presence of other neurological impairments. At the molecular level, resistance to AEDs may result from changes to molecules that act as targets for these drugs such as ion channels and from the upregulation of efflux drug transporters such as P-glycoprotein in response to seizures. Genetic differences between patients may contribute to a difference in the level of these changes, and thus contribute to pharmacoresistance. Current treatment options available to these patients include trials of the new AEDs, especially those with novel mechanisms of action, dietary modulation, vagus nerve stimulation and resective surgery. As the mechanisms underlying pharmacoresistance become better understood, future strategies might include inhibition of efflux transporters and design of drugs which act on altered targets. Identification of genetic markers that alter the pharmacology of certain drugs might allow for the prediction of responders and hence more rational prescribing of AEDs.

REFERENCES

Aicardi, J. (1990). Epilepsy in brain-injured children. *Dev Med Child Neurol* **32**, 191-202.

Amar, A.P., DeGiorgio, C.M., Tarver, W.B. and Apuzzo, M.L. (1999). Long-term multi-center experience with vagus nerve stimulation for intractable partial seizures: results of the XE5 trial. *Stereotact Funct Neurosurg* **73**, 104-108.

Andrade-Valenca, L.P., Valenca, M.M., Ribeiro, L.T., Matos, A.L., Sales, L.V., Velasco, T.R., Santos, A.C. and Leite, J.P. (2003). Clinical and neuroimaging features of good and poor seizure control patients with mesial temporal lobe epilepsy and hippocampal atrophy. *Epilepsia* **44**, 807-814.

Annegers, J.F., Hauser, W.A. and Elveback, L.R. (1979). Remission of seizures and relapse in patients with epilepsy. *Epilepsia* **20**, 729-737.

Aronica, E., Gorter, J.A., Jansen, G.H. *et al.* (2003). Expression and cellular distribution of multidrug transporter proteins in two major causes of medically intractable epilepsy: focal cortical dysplasia and glioneuronal tumors. *Neuroscience* **118**, 417-429.

Aronica, E., Gorter, J.A., Ramkema, M. *et al.* (2004). Expression and cellular distribution of multidrug resistance-related proteins in the hippocampus of patients with mesial temporal lobe epilepsy. *Epilepsia* **45**, 441-451.

Ballerini, P., Di Lorio, P., Ciccarelli R. *et al.* (2002). Glial cells express multiple ATP binding cassette proteins which are involved in ATP release. *NeurorReport* **13**, 1789-1792.

Bendayan, R., Lee, G. and Bendayan, M. (2002). Functional expression and localization of P-glycoprotein at the blood brain barrier. *Microsc Res Tech* **57**, 365-380.

Ben-Menachem, E. (1996). Modern management of epilepsy: Vagus nerve stimulation. *Baillieres Clin Neurol* **5**, 841-848.

Berg, A.T., Langfitt, J., Shinnar, S. *et al.* (2003). How long does it take for partial epilepsy to become intractable? *Neurology* **60**, 186-190.

Bouilleret, V., Loup, F., Kiener, T. *et al.* (2000). Early loss of interneurons and delayed subunit-specific changes in GABA(A)-receptor expression in a mouse model of mesial temporal lobe epilepsy. *Hippocampus* **10**, 305-324.

Briellmann, R., Berkovic, S., Syngeniotis, A. *et al.* (2002). Seizure-associated hippocampal volume loss: a longitudinal magnetic resonance study of temporal lobe epilepsy. *Ann Neurol* **51**, 641-644.

Brodie, M.J. (2004). Glasgow outcome studies: new horizons in the development of antiepileptic drugs: the search for new targets. A conference review. *Epilepsy Res* **60**, 96-97.

Brooks-Kayal, A.R., Shumate, M.D., Jin, H. *et al.* (1998). Selective changes in single cell GABA(A) receptor subunit expression and function in temporal lobe epilepsy. *Nat Med* **4**, 1166-1172.

Callen, D.F., Baker, E., Simmers, R.N. *et al.* (1987). Localization of the human multiple drug resistance gene, MDR1, to 7q21.1. *Hum Genet* **77**, 142-144.

Camfield, P.R., Camfield, C.S., Gordon, K. *et al.* (1997). If a first antiepileptic drug fails to control a child's epilepsy, what are the chances of success with the next drug? *J Pediatr* **31**, 821-824.

Camfield, P.R. and Camfield, C.S. (1994). The prognosis of childhood epilepsy. *Semin Pediatr Neurol* **1**, 102-110.

Ceulemans, B.P., Claes, L.R. and Lagae, L.G. (2004). Clinical correlations of mutations in the SCN1A gene: from febrile seizures to severe myoclonic epilepsy in infancy. *Pediatr Neurol* **30**, 236-243.

Cockerell, O.C., Johnson, A.L., Sander, J.W. and Shorvon, S.D. (1997). Prognosis of epilepsy: a review and further analysis of the first nine years of the British National General Practice Study of Epilepsy, a prospective population-based study. *Epilepsia* **38**, 31-46.

Cockerell, O.C., Johnson, A.L., Sander, J.W.A.S. *et al.* (1995). Remission of epilepsy: results from the National General Practice Study of Epilepsy. *Lancet* **346**, 140-144.

Coppola, G., Veggiotti, P., Cusmai, R., Bertoli, S., Cardinali, S., Dionisi-Vici, C., Elia, M., Lispi, M.L., Sarnelli, C., Tagliabue, A., Toraldo, C. and Pascotto, A. (2002). The ketogenic diet in children, adolescents and young adults with refractory epilepsy: an Italian multicentric experience. *Epilepsy Res* **48**, 221–227.

Cornford, E.M. (1999). Epilepsy and the blood brain barrier: endothelial cell responses to seizures. *Adv Neurol* **79**, 845-862.

Cuadrado, A. and Armijo, J.A. (2005). Beneficial interaction between vigabatrin and valproate against seizures induced by pentylenetetrazole in mice. *Pharmacol Res* **51**, 489-496.

Cunnane, S.C., Musa, K., Ryan, M.A., Whiting, S. and Fraser, D.D. (2002). Potential role of polyunsaturates in seizure protection achieved with the ketogenic diet. *Prostaglandins Leukot Essent Fatty Acids* **67**, 131–135.

Dahlin, M., Elfving, A., Ungerstedt, U. and Amark, P. (2005). The ketogenic diet influences the levels of excitatory and inhibitory amino acids in the CSF in children with refractory epilepsy. *Epilepsy Res* **64**, 115-125.

Dean, M., Rzhetsky, A. and Allikmets, R. (2001). The human ATP-binding cassette (ABC) transporter superfamily. *Genome Res* **11**, 1156-1166.

DeGiorgio, C., Heck, C., Bunch, S., Britton, J., Green, P., Lancman, M., Murphy, J., Olejniczak, P., Shih, J., Arrambide, S. and Soss, J. (2005). Vagus nerve stimulation for epilepsy: randomized comparison of three stimulation paradigms. *Neurology* **65**, 317-319.

Demeule, M., Régina, A., Jodoin, J. *et al.* (2002). Drug transport to the brain: key roles for the efflux pump P-glycoprotein in the blood-brain barrier. *Vasc Pharm* **38**, 339-348.

Depondt, C., Cavalleri, G.L., Shorvon, S.D., Wood, N.W., Sissodiya, S.M. and Goldstein, D.B. (2005). Association study of five sodium channel genes in epilepsy and antiepileptic drug response. *Epilepsia* **46(Suppl)**, S90.

D'Giano, C., Sevlever, G. and Lazarowski, A. *et al.* (1997). Expression of P-glycoprotein and related proteins in brain of patients with refractory temporal-lobe epilepsy (TLE). *Epilepsia* **38 (Suppl 8)**, S87.

Dicato, M., Duhem, C., Pauly, M. *et al.* (1997). Multidrug resistance: molecular and clinical aspects. *Cytokines Cell Mol Ther* **3**, 91-100.

Dietzmann, K., Bossanyi, P.V. and Franke, D.S. (1994). Expression of P-glycoprotein as a multidrug resistance gene product in human reactive astrocytes and astrocytoma. *Zentralbl Pathol* **140**, 149-153.

Dombrowski, S.M., Desai, S.Y., Marroni, M. *et al.* (2001). Overexpression of multidrug resistance genes in endothelial cells from patients with refractory epilepsy. *Epilepsia* **42**, 1501-1506.

Eagles, D.A., Boyd, S.J., Kotak, A. an Allan, F. (2003). Calorie restriction of a high-carbohydrate diet elevates the threshold of PTZ-induced seizures to values equal to those seen with a ketogenic diet. *Epilepsy Res* **54**, 41–52.

Ellerkmann, R.K., Remy, S., Chen, J. *et al.* (2003). Molecular and functional changes in voltage-dependent Na(+) channels following pilocarpine-induced status epilepticus in rat dentate granule cells. *Neuroscience* **119**, 323-333.

Elwes, R.D., Johnson, A.L., Shorvon, S.D. and Reynolds, E.H. (1984). The prognosis for seizure control in newly diagnosed epilepsy. *N Engl J Med* **311**, 944-947.

Engel, J. (1987). Update on surgical treatment of the epilepsies. In: Engel, J. (Ed), *Surgical treatment of epilepsies*. Raven Press, New York pp32-48.

Forsgren, L. (1995). Epidemiology of intractable epilepsy in adults. In: Johannessen, S.I., Gram, L., Sillanpaa, M. *et al.* (Eds), *Intractable epilepsy*. Wrightson Biomedical Publishing, Petersfield, UK, pp. 25-40.

Freeman, J., Vining, E., Pillas, D., Pryzik, P., Casey, J. and Kelly, M. (1998). The efficacy of the ketogenic diet-1998: a prospective evaluation of intervention in 150 children. *Pediatrics* **102**, 1358–1363.

Freeman, J.M. and Vining, E.P.G. (1999). Seizures decrease rapidly after fasting: preliminary studies of the ketogenic diet. *Arch Pediatr Adolesc Med* **153**, 946–949.

French, J.A. *et al.* (2004). Efficacy and tolerability of the new antiepileptic drugs II: treatment of refractory epilepsy: report of the Therapeutics and Technology Assessment Subcommittee and Quality Standards Subcommittee of the American Academy of Neurology and the American Epilepsy Society. *Neurology* **62**, 1261-1273.

French, J.A., Kugler, A.R., Robbins, J.L. *et al.* (2003). Dose-response trial of pregabalin adjunctive therapy in patients with partial seizures. *Neurology* **60**, 1631-1637.

Fritschy, J.M., Kiener, T., Bouilleret, V. *et al.* (1999). GABAergic neurons and GABA(A)-receptors in temporal lobe epilepsy. *Neurochem Int* **34**, 435-445.

Fuerst, D., Shah, A. and Watson, C. (2003). Hippocampal sclerosis is a progressive disorder: a longitudinal volumetric MRI study. *Ann Neurol* **53**, 413-416.

Gao, B., Hagenbuch, B. and Kullak-Ublick, G.A. *et al.* (2000). Organic anion-transporting polypeptides mediate transport of opioid peptides across blood-brain barrier. *J Pharmacol Exp Ther* **294**. 73-79.

Gibbs, J.P., Adeyeye, M.C., Yang, Z. *et al.* (2004). Valproic acid uptake by bovine brain microvessel endothelial cells: role of active efflux transport. *Epilepsy Res* **58**, 53-66.

Gilby, K.L., Da Silva, A.G. and McIntyre, D.C. (2005). Differential GABA(A) subunit expression following status epilepticus in seizure-prone and seizure-resistant rats: a putative mechanism for refractory drug response. *Epilepsia* **46 (Suppl 5)**, S3-S9.

Golden, P.L. and Pardridge, W.M. (1999). P-glycoprotein on astrocytes foot processes of unfixed isolated human brain capillaries. *Brain Res* **819**, 143-146.

Gottesman, M.M., Fojo, T. and Bates, S.E. (2002). Multidrug resistance in cancer: role of ATP-dependent transporters. *Nat Rev Cancer* **2**, 48-58.

Handforth, A., DeGiorgio, C.M., Schachter, S.C., Uthman, B.M., Naritoku, D.K., Tecoma, E.S., Henry, T.R., Collins, S.D., Vaugh, B.V., Gilmartin, R.C., Labar, D.R., Morris, G.L. III, Salinsky, M.C., Osorio, I., Ristanovic, R.K., Labiner, D.M., Jones, J.C., Murphy, J.V., Ney, G.C. and Wheless, J.W. (1998). Vagus nerve stimulation therapy for partial-onset seizures: a randomized active-control trial. *Neurology* **51**, 48-55.

Hauser, W.A. (1992). The natural history of drug resistant epilepsy: epidemiologic considerations. *Epilepsy Res Suppl* **5**, 25-28.

Hemingway, C., Freeman, J.M., Pillas, D.J. and Pyzik, P.L. (2001). The ketogenic diet: a 3- to 6-year follow-up of 150 children enrolled prospectively. *Pediatrics* **108**, 898–905.

Hung, C.C., Tai, J.J., Lin, C.J., Lee, M.J. and Liou, H.H. (2005). Complex haplotypic effects of the ABCB1 gene on epilepsy treatment response. *Pharmacogenomics* **6**, 411-417.

Iannetti, P., Spalice, A. and Parisi, P. (2005). Calcium-channel blocker verapamil administration in prolonged and refractory status epilepticus. *Epilepsia* **46**, 967-969.

Isom, L.L. (2002). Beta subunits: players in neuronal hyperexcitability? *Novartis Found Symp* **241**, 124-138.

Jeong, S.W., Lee, S.K., Hong, K.S., Kim, K.K., Chung, C.K. and Kim, H. (2005). Prognostic factors for the surgery for mesial temporal lobe epilepsy: longitudinal analysis. *Epilepsia* **46**, 1273-1279.

Jones, D.M., Esmaeil, N., Maren, S. *et al.* (2002). Characterization of pharmacoresistance to benzodiazepines in the rat Li-pilocarpine model of status epilepticus. *Epilepsy Res* **50**, 301-112.

Jutila, L., Immonen, A., Mervaala, E., Partanen, J., Partanen, K., Puranen, M., Kalviainen, R., Alafuzoff, I., Hurskainen, H., Vapalahti, M. and Ylinen, A. (2002). Long term outcome of temporal lobe epilepsy surgery: analyses of 140 consecutive patients. *J Neurol Neurosurg Psychiatry* **73**, 486-494.

Kamiya, K., Kaneda, M., Sugawara, T., Mazaki, E., Okamura, N., Montal, M., Makita, N., Tanaka, M., Fukushima, K., Fujiwara, T., Inoue, Y. and Yamakawa, K.A. (2004). Nonsense mutation of the sodium channel gene SCN2A in a patient with intractable epilepsy and mental decline. *J Neurosci* **24**, 2690-2698.

Katyal, N.G., Koehler, A.N., McGhee, B., Foley, C.M. and Crumrine, P.K. (2000). The ketogenic diet in refractory epilepsy: the experience of Children's Hospital of Pittsburgh. *Clin Pediatr* **39**, 153–159.

Kim, W.J., Park, S.C., Lee, S.J. *et al.* (1999). The prognosis for control of seizures with medications in patients with MRI evidence for mesial temporal sclerosis. *Epilepsia* **40**, 290-293.

Klein, I., Sarkadi, B. and Váradi, A. (1999). An inventory of the human ABC proteins. *Biochim Biophys Acta* **1461**, 237-262.

Kossoff, E.H., Krauss, G.L., McGrogan, J.R. and Freeman, J.M. (2003). Efficacy of the Atkins diet as a therapy for intractable epilepsy. *Neurology* **61**, 1789–1791.

Kumlien, E., Doss, R.C. and Gates, J.R. (2002). Treatment outcome in patients with mesial temporal sclerosis. *Seizure* **11**, 413-417.

Kwan, P. and Brodie, M.J. (2000). Early identification of refractory epilepsy. *N Engl J Med* **342**, 314-319.

Kwan, P., Brodie, M.J. (2001). Effectiveness of first antiepileptic drug. *Epilepsia* **42**, 1255-1260.

Kwan, P. and Brodie, M.J. (2005). Potential role of drug transporters in the pathogenesis of medically intractable epilepsy. Epilepsia. 2005; **46**, 224-35

Labar, D., Murphy, J. and Tecoma, E. (1999). Vagus nerve stimulation for medication-resistant generalized epilepsy. E04 VNS Study Group. *Neurology* **52**, 1510-1512

Labar, D., Nikolov, B., Tarver, B. and Fraser, R. (1998). Vagus nerve stimulation for symptomatic generalized epilepsy: a pilot study. *Epilepsia*. **39**, 201-205.

Langmann, T., Mauerer, R., Zahn, A. *et al.* (2003). Real-time reverse transcription-PCR expression profiling of the complete human ATP-binding cassette transporter superfamily in various tissues. *Clin Chem* **49**, 230-238.

Lardizabal, D.V., Jacobson, B., Ying, Z. *et al.* (2003). Multidrug resistance-1 (MDR1) protein expression in Rasmussen encephalitis. *Epilepsia* **44(Suppl 9)**, S35-S36.

Lazarowski, A., Lubieniecki, F., Camarero, H.T. *et al.* (2004). Multidrug resistance proteins in tuberous sclerosis and refractory epilepsy. *Pediatr Neurol* **102**, 30-36.

Lee, G., Dallas, S., Hong, M. and Bendayan, R. (2001). Drug transporters in the central nervous system: brain barriers and brain parenchyma consideration. *Pharmacol Rev* **53**, 569-596.

Lehericy, S., Semah, F., Hasboun, D., Dormont, D., Clemenceau, S., Granat, O., Marsault, C. and Baulac, M. (1997). Temporal lobe epilepsy with varying severity: MRI study of 222 patients. *Neuroradiology* **39**, 788-796.

Löscher, W. and Schmidt, D. (2004). New horizons in the development of antiepileptic drugs: the search for new targets. *Epilepsy Res* **60**, 77-159.

Loup, F., Wieser, H.G., Yonekawa, Y. *et al.* (2000). Selective alterations in GABA$_A$ receptor subtypes in human temporal lobe epilepsy. *J Neurosci* **20**, 5401-5419.

Luer, M.S., Hamani, C., Dujovny, M. *et al.* (1999). Saturable transport of gabapentin at the blood-brain barrier. *Neurol Res* **21**, 559-562.

Lundgren, J., Amark, P., Blennow, G., Stromblad, L.G. and Wallstedt, L. (1998). Vagus nerve stimulation in 16 children with refractory epilepsy. *Epilepsia* **39**, 809-813.

Luszczki, J.J., Andres, M.M. and Czuczwar, S.J. (2005). Synergistic interaction of gabapentin and oxcarbazepine in the mouse maximal electroshock seizure model—an isobolographic analysis. *Eur J Pharmacol* **15**, 54-61.

Lynch, B.A., Lambeng, N., Nocka, K. *et al.* (2004). The synaptic vesicle protein SV2A is the binding site for the antiepileptic drug levetiracetam. *Proc Natl Acad Sci USA* **101**, 9861-9866.

Matsumoto, T., Tani, E., Kaba, K. *et al.* (1991). Expression of P-glycoprotein in human glioma cell lines and surgical glioma specimens. *J Neurosurg* **74**, 460-466.

Maydell, B.V., Wyllie, E., Akhtar, N., Kotagal, P., Powaski, K., Cook, K., Weinstock, A. and Rothner, A.D. (2001). Efficacy of the ketogenic diet in focal versus generalized seizures. *Pediatr Neurol* **25**, 208–212.

McIntosh, A.M., Kalnins, R.M., Mitchell, L.A., Fabinyi, G.C., Briellmann, R.S. and Berkovic, S.F. (2004). Temporal lobectomy: long-term seizure outcome, late recurrence and risks for seizure recurrence. *Brain* **127**, 2018-2030.

Muller, B. (2001). Psychological approaches to the prevention and inhibition of nocturnal epileptic seizures: a meta-analysis of 70 case studies. *Seizure* **10**, 13-33.

Nishimura, T., Schwarzer, C., Gasser, E., Kato, N., Vezzani, A. and Sperk, G. (2005). Altered expression of GABA(a) and GABA(b) receptor subunit mRNAs in the hippocampus after kindling and electrically induced status epilepticus. *Neuroscience* **134**, 691-704.

Owen, A., Pirmohamed, M., Tettey, J.N. *et al.* (2001). Carbamazepine is not a substrate for P-glycoprotein. *Br J Clin Pharmacol* **51**, 345-349.

Pardridge, W.M., Golden, P.L., Kang, Y.S. *et al.* (1997). Brain microvascular and astrocyte localization of P-glycoprotein. *J Neurochem* **68**, 1278-1285.

Patsalos, P.N. and Perucca, E. (2003). Clinically important drug interactions in epilepsy: general features and interactions between antiepileptic drugs. *Lancet Neurol* **2**, 347-356.

Penry, J.K. and Dean, J.C. (1990). Prevention of intractable partial seizures by intermittent vagal stimulation in humans: preliminary results. *Epilepsia* **31 (Suppl 2)**, S40-S43.

Perucca, E. (1998). Pharmacoresistance in epilepsy: how should it be defined? *CNS Drugs* **10**, 171-179.

Pirker, S., Schwarzer, C., Czech, T., Baumgartner, C., Pockberger, H., Maier, H., Hauer, B., Sieghart, W., Furtinger, S. and Sperk, G. (2003). Increased expression of GABA$_A$ receptor beta-subunits in the hippocampus of patients with temporal lobe epilepsy. *J Neuropathol Exp Neurol* **62**, 820-834.

Potschka H, and Löscher W. (2001a). In vivo evidence for P-glycoprotein-mediated transport of phenytoin at the blood-brain barrier of rats. Epilepsia 2001; **42**: 1231-40

Potschka H, and Löscher W. (2001b). Multidrug resistance-associated protein is involved in the regulation of extracellular levels of phenytoin in the brain. Neuroreport 2001; **12**: 2387-2389.

Potschka H, Volk HA, and Löscher W. (2004). Pharmacoresistance and expression of multidrug transporter P-glycoprotein in kindled rats. Neuroreport 2004;15: 1657-61

Potschka H, Fedrowitz M and, Löscher W. (2001). P-Glycoprotein and multidrug resistance-associated protein are involved in the regulation of extracellular levels of the major antiepileptic drug carbamazepine in the brain. Neuroreport 2001;12: 3557-60

Potschka H, Fedrowitz M and, Löscher W. (2002). P-Glycoprotein-mediated efflux of phenobarbital, lamotrigine, and felbamate at the blood-brain barrier: evidence from microdialysis experiments in rats. Neurosci Lett 2002;327: 173-6

Potschka H, Fedrowitz M and, Löscher W. (2003a). Multidrug resistance protein MRP2 contributes to blood-brain barrier function and restricts antiepileptic drug activity. J Pharmacol Exp Ther 2003;306: 124-31

Potschka, H., Fedrowitz, M. and Löscher, W. (2003b). Brain access and anticonvulsant efficacy of carbamazepine, lamotrigine, and felbamate in ABCC2/MRP2-deficient TR- rats. Epilepsia 44, 1479-1486.

Potschka, H., Baltes, S. and Löscher, W. (2004). Inhibition of multidrug transporters by verapamil or probenecid does not alter blood-brain barrier penetration of levetiracetam in rats. Epilepsy Res 58, 85-91.

Privitera, M.D., Welty, T.E., Ficker, D.M. and Welge., J. (2002). Vagus nerve stimulation for partial seizures. Cochrane Database Syst Rev (1), CD002896.

Ramaratnam, S., Baker, G.A. and Goldstein, L. (2003). Psychological treatments for epilepsy. Cochrane Database Syst Rev (4), CD002029.

Rao, V.V., Dahlheimer, J.L., Bardgett, M.E. et al. (1999). Choroid plexus epithelial expression of MDR1 P-glycoprotein and multidrug resistance-associated protein contribute to the blood-cerebrospinal-fluid drug permeability barrier. Proc Natl Acad Sci USA 96, 3900-3905.

Redecker, C., Luhmann, H.J., Hagemann, G. et al. (2000). Differential downregulation of GABA_A receptor subunits in widespread brain regions in the freeze-lesion model of focal cortical malformations. J Neurosci 20, 5045-5053.

Regesta, G. and Tanganelli, P. (1999). Clinical aspects and biological bases of drug-resistant epilepsies. Epilepsy Res 34, 109-122.

Remy, S., Gabriel, S., Urban, B.W. et al. (2003). A novel mechanism underlying drug resistance in chronic epilepsy. Ann Neurol 53, 469-479.

Remy, S., Urban, B.W., Elger, C.E. et al. (2003). Anticonvulsant pharmacology of voltage-gated Na+ channels in hippocampal neurons of control and chronically epileptic rats. Eur J Neurosci 17, 2648-2658.

Rizzi, M., Caccia, S., Guiso, G. et al. (2002). Limbic seizures induce P-glycoprotein in rodent brain: functional implications for pharmacoresistance. J Neurosci 22, 5833-5839.

Rodriguez, I., Abernethy, D.R. and Woosley, R.L. (1999). P-glycoprotein in clinical cardiology. Circulation 99, 472-474.

Rowan, A.J., Overweg, J., Sadikoglu, S., Binnie, C.D., Nagelkerke, N.J. and Hunteler, E. (1980). Seizure prognosis in long-stay mentally subnormal epileptic patients:inter-rater EEG and clinical studies. Epilepsia 21, 219-225.

Rudolph, U. and Möhler, H. (2004). Analysis of GABA(A) receptor function and dissection of the pharmacology of benzodiazepines and general anesthetics through mouse genetics. Ann Rev Pharmacol Toxicol 44, 475-498.

Salinsky, M.C., Uthman, B.M., Ristanovic, R.K., Wernicke, J.F. and Tarver, W.B. (1996). Vagus nerve stimulation for the treatment of medically intractable seizures. Results of a 1-year open-extension trial. Vagus Nerve Stimulation Study Group. Arch Neurol 53, 1176-1180.

Schinkel, A.H., Smit, J.J.M., van Tellingen, O. *et al.* (1994). Disruption of the mouse mdr1a P-glycoprotein gene leads to a deficiency in the blood-brain barrier and to increased sensitivity to drugs. *Cell* **77**, 491-502.

Schinkel, A.H. (1997). The physiological function of drug-transporting P-glycoproteins. *Semin Cancer Biol* **8**, 161-170.

Schlanger, S., Shinitzky, M. and Yam, D. (2002). Diet enriched with omega-3 fatty acids alleviates convulsion symptoms in epilepsy patients. *Epilepsia* **43**, 103–104.

Schmid-Schonbein, C. (1998). Improvement of seizure control by psychological methods in patients with intractable epilepsies. *Seizure* **7**, 261-270.

Schmidt, D. and Löscher, W. (2005). Drug resistance in epilepsy: putative neurobiologic and clinical mechanisms. *Epilepsia* **46**, 858-877.

Seegers, U., Potschka, H. and Löscher, W. (2002). Transient increase of P-glycoprotein expression in endothelium and parenchyma of limbic brain regions in the kainate model of temporal lobe epilepsy. *Epilepsy Res* **51**, 257-268.

Seelig, A. (1998). A general pattern for substrate recognition by P-glycoprotein. *Eur J Biochem* **251**, 252-261.

Semah, F., Picot, M.C., Adam, C. *et al.* (1998). Is the underlying cause of epilepsy a major prognostic factor for recurrence? *Neurology* **51**, 1256-1262.

Sharom, J.F. (1997). The P-glycoprotein efflux pump: how does it transport drugs? *J Membrane Biol* **160**, 161-175.

Shorvon, S.D., Lowenthal, A., Janz, D., Bielen, E. and Loiseau, P. (2000). Multicenter double-blind, randomized, placebo-controlled trial of levetiracetam as add-on therapy in patients with refractory partial seizures. European Levetiracetam Study Group. *Epilepsia* **41**, 1179-1186.

Shorvon, S.D. and Reynolds, E.H. (1982). Early prognosis of epilepsy. *BMJ (Clin Res Ed)*. **285**, 1699-1701.

Shorvon, S.D. and Sander, J.W.A.S. (1986). Temporal patterns of remission and relapse in seizures of patients with epilepsy. In: Schmidt D and Morselli, P.L. (Eds), *Intractable epilepsy: experimental and clinical aspects*. Raven Press, New York, pp. 3-24.

Siddiqui, A., Kerb, R., Weale, M.E., Brinkmann, U., Smith, A., Goldstein, D.B., Wood, N.W. and Sisodiya, S.M. (2003). Association of multidrug resistance in epilepsy with a polymorphism in the drug-transporter gene ABCB1. *N Engl J Med* **348**, 1442-1448.

Sieghart, W. and Sperk, G. (2002). Subunit composition, distribution and function of GABA(A) receptor subtypes. *Curr Top Med Chem* **2**, 795-816.

Sillanpää, M. (1993). Remission of seizures and predictors of intractability in long-term follow-up. *Epilepsia* **34**, 930-936.

Sillanpää, M., Jalava, M. and Shinnar, S. (1999). Epilepsy syndromes in patients with childhood-onset seizures in Finland. *Pediatr Neurol* **21**, 533-537.

Sills, G.J., Kwan, P., Butler, E. *et al.* (2002). P-glycoprotein-mediated efflux of antiepileptic drugs: preliminary studies in mdr1a knockout mice. *Epilepsy Behav* **3**, 427-432.

Sills, G.J., Butler, E., Thompson, G.G. and Brodie, M.J. (2004). Pharmacodynamic interaction studies with topiramate in the pentylenetetrazol and maximal electroshock seizure models. *Seizure* **13**, 287-295.

Sills, G.J., Mohanraj, R., Butler, E., McCrindle, S., Collier, L., Wilson, E.A. and Brodie, M.J. (2005). Lack of association between the C3435T polymorphism in the human multidrug resistance (MDR1) gene and response to antiepileptic drug treatment. *Epilepsia* **46**, 643-647.

Silverman, J.A. (1999). Multidrug-resistance transporters. *Pharmaceut Biotech* **12**, 353-386.

Sisodiya, S.M., Heffernan, J. and Squier, M.V. (1999). Over-expression of P-glycoprotein in malformations of cortical development. *Neuroreport* **10**, 3437-3441.

Sisodiya, S.M., Lin, W.R., Harding, B.N. *et al.* (2002). Drug resistance in epilepsy: expression of drug resistance proteins in common causes of refractory epilepsy. *Brain* **125**, 22-31.

Sisodiya, S.M., Martinian, L., Scheffer, G.L., van der Valk, P., Cross, J.H., Scheper, R.J.,Harding, B.N. and Thom, M. (2003). Major vault protein, a marker of drug resistance, is upregulated in refractory epilepsy. *Epilepsia* **44**, 1388-1396.

Sofijanov, N.G. (1982). Clinical evolution and prognosis of childhood epilepsies. *Epilepsia* **23**, 61-69.

Spencer, S.S., Berg, A.T., Vickrey, B.G., Sperling, M.R., Bazil, C.W., Shinnar, S., Langfitt, J.T., Walczak, T.S. and Pacia S.V. (2005). Multicenter Study of Epilepsy Surgery. Predicting long-term seizure outcome after resective epilepsy surgery: the multicenter study. *Neurology* **65(6)**, 912-918.

Sperk, G., Schwarzer, C., Tsunashima, K. *et al.* (1998). Expression of GABA(A) receptor subunits in the hippocampus of the rat after kainic acid-induced seizures. *Epilepsy Res* **32**, 129-139.

Sperling, M.R. (2004). The consequences of uncontrolled epilepsy. *CNS Spectrums* **9**, 98-101, 106-109.

Stafstrom, C.E. (2004). Dietary approaches to epilepsy treatment: old and new options on the menu. *Epilepsy Curr* **4**, 215-222.

Stafstrom, C.E. (2001). Effects of fatty acids and ketones on neuronal excitability: implications for epilepsy and its treatment. In: Mostofsky, D.I., Yehuda, S. and Salem, N. Jr. (Eds), *Fatty acids: physiological and behavioral functions. Vol. 2001.* Humana Press, Totowa, NJ, pp. 273–290.

Stephen, L.J., Kwan, P. and Brodie, M.J. (2001). Does the cause of localisation-related epilepsy influence the response to anticpileptic drug treatment? *Epilepsia* **42**, 357-362.

Summers, M.A., Moore, J.L. and McAuley, J.W. (2004). Use of verapamil as a potential p-glycoprotein inhibitor in a patient with refractory epilepsy. *Ann Pharmacother* **38**, 1631-1634.

Sutula, T.P., Hagen, J. and Pitkänen, A. (2003). Do epileptic seizures damage the brain? *Curr Opin Neurol* **16**, 189-195.

Tan, N.C., Heron, S.E., Scheffer, I.E., Pelekanos, J.T., McMahon, J.M., Vears, D.F., Mulley, J.C. and Berkovic, S.F. (2004). Failure to confirm association of a polymorphism in ABCB1 with multidrug-resistant epilepsy. *Neurology* **63**, 1090-1092.

Taylor, E.M. (2002). The impact of efflux transporters in the brain on the development of drugs for CNS disorders. *Clin Pharmacokinet* **41**, 81-92.

Tellez-Zenteno, J.F., Dhar, R. and Wiebe, S. (2005). Long-term seizure outcomes following epilepsy surgery: a systematic review and meta-analysis. *Brain* **128**, 1188-1198.

Terry, R., Tarver, W.B. and Zabara, J. (1990). An implantable neurocybernetic prosthesis system. *Epilepsia* **31(Suppl 2)**, S33-S37.

The Vagus Nerve Stimulation Study Group. (1995). A randomized controlled trial of chronic vagus nerve stimulation for treatment of medically intractable seizures. *Neurology* **45**, 224-230.

Tishler, D.M., Weinberg, K.I., Hinton, D.R. *et al.* (1995). MD1 gene expression in brain of patients with medically intractable epilepsy. *Epilepsia* **36**, 1-6.

Uauy, R. and Mena, P. (2001). Lipids and neurodevelopment. *Nutr Rev* **59**, S34–S58.

Uthman, B.M., Wilder, B.J., Hammond, E.J. and Reid, S.A. (1990). Efficacy and safety of vagus nerve stimulation in patients with complex partial seizures. *Epilepsia* **31(Suppl 2)**, S44-S50.

Van Paesschen, W., Duncan, J.S., Stevens, J.M. and Connelly, A. (1997). Etiology and early prognosis of newly diagnosed partial seizures in adults: a quantitative hippocampal MRI study. *Neurology* **49**, 753-757.

Van Veen, H.W. and Konings, W.N. (1997). Multidrug transporters from bacteria to man: similarities in structure and function. *Semin Cancer Biol* **8**, 183-191.

Vining, E., Freeman, J., Ballaban-Gil, K., Camfield, C., Camfield, P., Holmes, G., Shinnar, S., Shuman, R., Trevathan, E. and Wheless, J. (1998). A multicenter study of the efficacy of the ketogenic diet. *Arch Neurol* **55**, 1433–1437.

Volk, H.A., Potschka, H. and Löscher, W. (2004a). Increased expression of the multidrug transporter P-glycoprotein in limbic brain regions after amygdala-kindled seizures in rats. *Epilepsy Res* **58**, 67-79.

Volk, H.A., Burkhardt, K., Potschka, H., Chen, J., Becker, A. and Löscher, W. (2004b). Neuronal expression of the drug efflux transporter P-glycoprotein in the rat hippocampus after limbic seizures. *Neuroscience* **123**, 751-759.

Voskuyl, R.A., Vreugdenhil, M., Kang, J.X. and Leaf, A. (1998). Anticonvulsant effect of polyunsaturated fatty acids in rats, using the cortical stimulation model. *Eur J Pharmacol* **341**, 145–152.

Vreugdenhil, M., Bruehl, C., Voskuyl, R.A., Kang, J.X., Leaf, A. and Wadman, W.J. (1996). Polyunsaturated fatty acids modulate sodium and calcium currents in CA1 neurons. *Proc Natl Acad Sci USA* **93**, 12559–12563.

Vreugdenhil, M., Vanveelen, C.W.M, Vanrijen PC *et al.* (1998). Effect of valproic acid on sodium currents in cortical neurons from patients with pharmaco-resistant temporal lobe epilepsy. *Epilepsy Res* **32**, 309-320.

Vreugdenhil, M. and Wadman, W.J. (1999). Modulation of sodium currents in rat CA1 neurons by carbamazepine and valproate after kindling epileptogenesis. *Epilepsia* **40**, 1512-1522.

Wilder, R.M. (1921). The effects of ketonemia on the course of epilepsy. *Mayo Clin Proc* **2**, 307–308.

Xiao, Y-F. and Li, X. (1999). Polyunsaturated fatty acids modify mouse hippocampal neuronal excitability during excitotoxic or convulsant stimulation. *Brain Res* **846**, 112–121.

Yamada, K.A., Rensing, N. and Thio, L.L. (2000). Ketogenic diet reduces hypoglycemia-induced neuronal death in young rats. *Neurosci Lett* **385**, 210-214.

Yehuda, S., Carasso, R.L. and Mostofsky, D.I. (1994). Essential fatty acid preparation (SR-3) raises the seizure threshold in rats. *Eur J Pharmacol* **254**, 193–198.

Yoon, H.H., Kwon, H.L., Mattson, R.H., Spencer, D.D. and Spencer, S.S. (2003). Long-term seizure outcome in patients initially seizure-free after resective epilepsy surgery. *Neurology* **61**, 445-450.

Yudkoff, M., Daikhin, Y., Nissim, I., Horyn, O., Lazarow, A., Luhovyy, B., Wehrli, S. and Nissim, I. (2005). Response of brain amino acid metabolism to ketosis. *Neurochem Int* **47**, 119-128.

Zhang, L., Ong, W.Y. and Lee, T. (1999). Induction of P-glycoprotein expression in astrocytes following intracerebroventricular kainate injections. *Exp Brain Res* **126**, 509-516.

Zimprich, F., Sunder-Plassmann, R., Stogmann, E., Gleiss, A., Dal-Bianco, A., Zimprich, A., Plumer, S., Baumgartner, C. and Mannhalter, C. (2004). Association of an ABCB1 gene haplotype with pharmacoresistance in temporal lobe epilepsy. *Neurology* **63**, 1087-1089.

9

The Patient's Perspective

SUSAN C. USISKIN

The National Hospital for Neurology & Neurosurgery,
Queen Square, London, UK

INTRODUCTION

This chapter aims to consider the prospect of seizure freedom from the patient's view point. During recent years the advent of many new anti-epileptic drugs for the treatment of epilepsy has meant that freedom from seizures is now a real possibility in a greater number of patients than was previously the case. With increasing awareness of the risks of mortality and morbidity for the patient, freedom from seizures is an important treatment goal for both the clinician and the patient and this will be discussed, along with the possible costs of seizure freedom, side effect issues, CNS effects and other possible changes including emotional, psychological and possibly neuropsychiatric ones. Treatment for epilepsy may also affect cognition, quality of life and the patient's libido. What sacrifices patients are willing to make for the sake of being free from seizures varies enormously and, as a clinical counsellor for patients with severe epilepsy, I am constantly brought up against this question and I am struck by the broad range of patients willing to accept these changes.

Much depends on the patient's own perspective of epilepsy as a stigma-tising disorder. Stigma may be defined as a condition that renders a person unacceptably different from his or her peers or social group. There are often public perceptions of epilepsy which patients share and those patients who feel most stigmatised by the disorder are often willing to make the greatest sacrifices when it comes to potential treatments. These and other social aspects of seizure freedom will be discussed. In recent years, we also have the option of epilepsy surgery which offers the only potential cure for the causes of seizures and this form of treatment is increasingly offered where it is thought to be appropriate (see also Chapter 5 – this book).

As a person with epilepsy myself, diagnosed while I was still at school, I have several decades of personal experience in living with severe and frequent seizures throughout various phases of my life and the implications of this will also be discussed in relation to what seizure freedom and the lack of it may mean in pregnancy, child birth and the experience of being a mother with epilepsy.

COMMON MISCONCEPTIONS CONCERNING EPILEPSY

- The association of epilepsy with mental illness and mental handicap.
- The assumption that seizures themselves (i.e. single seizures) cause brain damage.
- Presumed inheritance (i.e. regardless of aetiology, etc.).
- Epilepsy is for life (no remission possible).
- Seizures are 100% controllable by medication (and if they do occur you are under-medicated!).

TREATMENT GOALS

The clinician

People with epilepsy have a mortality rate which is two to three times higher than that of the general population. It also carries a morbidity rate which may include major and minor injuries, as well as psychosocial difficulties and most clinicians will want to protect patients with seizures from these possible consequences.

Clinicians may attempt a number of medical treatments until they are satisfied that the best control of the patient's condition has been achieved with minimum cost to the patient in terms of unpleasant side effects. The hope will be to achieve this within the first few years of diagnosis and therefore afford each individual patient with maximum utility of their life with minimum costs to them in terms of sacrifices.

The patient

It is my experience, both as a patient with epilepsy myself and with many years of clinical experience talking to patients referred to me, that control of seizures is enormously important and is a treatment goal for all patients. I have personal experience of treatment with many different anti-epileptic drugs over the years in the quest for better control of my seizures only to find that they have proven to be ineffective or had unacceptable side effects which limited their clinical use for me. In my own case as I was diagnosed long before brain scanning was available as a diagnostic tool for the causes of epilepsy; I think it is fair to conclude that some of these drugs would not have been used for me if it had been diagnosed some decades later. It is indeed fortunate that patients investigated and diagnosed today will, in the main, be tried on targeted treatments for their own differential diagnosis. This means for a surprising number of patients that now they stand a better chance of becoming seizure-free in a shorter period of time than was the case in the past. This is an important development in the treatment of epilepsy for a number of reasons and these may include the patient being able to understand more about the clinical reasons why they have developed epilepsy in the first place.

During recent years the possibility of surgical treatment for persistent and drug resistant seizures offers some patients the very real possibility of a cure. As such patients are very carefully screened before it is decided whether or not they are suited to surgical treatment and it is possible for their neurologist to discuss with them what their individual odds of becoming seizure-free are in increasingly accurate terms. For those patients who undergo successful surgery for epilepsy it is important to consider what being free from seizures will mean to them individually.

SEIZURE FREEDOM – A POTENTIAL PROBLEM?

It may seem strange that the possibility of seizure freedom in a patient for whom long years of intractable seizures are ultimately exchanged for complete, or near-complete control, could possibly be a problem. This however represents a considerable emotional adjustment on the part of some patients, especially for those whose lives have been dominated by problematic epilepsy.

This type of dramatic improvement as a result of surgery (or improved medical control) may bring new challenges for some. Changes may include eventual loss of financial benefits, alteration in the level of expectations both from the patients and their families viewpoint and there may be adjustment problems experienced both by the patient, their family and friends. Confusion as to what to expect and changes in the level of protection for the patient are common, as are tense anticipations regarding the real possibility of independent living, driving, going to college, training and employment. Some of these notions may be difficult for the patient to face up to at first and it is important that good communication with those who understand these issues is part of their clinical follow-up which will need to look at their new found state in a holistic and balanced way. In those for whom it is clear that the change that they have undergone is becoming a problem, counselling is likely to be helpful.

Over the years I have counselled many patients who have undergone such life experiences as a result of achieving better or complete control of their seizures, and I am aware that the adjustment for some, particularly those who have been over- protected by well-meaning families, may be difficult. I have even known patients who, following epilepsy surgery which has rendered them seizure-free for more than 12 months, have opted to stay on their medication, even when their clinician has discussed the possibility of reducing and eventually coming off their drugs altogether. It is true that these particular patients have been in the minority but they do exist and it is important that they receive the appropriate help to enable them to adjust successfully over time to what for them is a new way of living.

People with epilepsy who know they may not be free from seizures and still manage to engage with life are less likely to manifest this sort of adjustment problem. For them relative or complete freedom from seizures will come as a tremendous bonus and a platform from which they can take their life forward in a truly positive manner.

WOMEN AND SEIZURE FEEDOM

There are many special issues relating to women and particular reasons why the possibility of better treatments maybe so poignant in relation to their life. When I think of what I went through myself many years ago with my two pregnancies and thereafter being responsible for bringing up my two children, I wish that I had been then in as relatively good health as I am today. Being a prospective parent and then mother of small children was fraught with difficulties, and when I look back on it now I see the many improvements that have been achieved for me through surgery and new drug treatments.

At the time when I embarked on my first pregnancy, the frequent seizures from which I suffered were treated with ever increasing amounts of several different anti-epileptic drugs. At that time, I was not warned of the effects my medication may have on the development of my babies and luckily my son was unaffected but when our daughter was born this marked the beginning of an intensely traumatic few years for my husband and myself. Our daughter showed clear signs of the effects of polytherapy and was critically ill for the first two years of her life. At that time we were not counselled on the potential effects of the medication I was taking, as patients usually are today. When I think back over these experiences related to my condition, I marvel at the fact that we managed to get through this critical phase of bringing up small children at all.

I was extremely fortunate in having a very supportive and practical husband who took an active part in helping and covering for me when I was too unwell to look after our children. If he was not around, I would never bathe my small son or daughter until he got home in case I had a seizure and risked my children coming to some harm through this. It was very important at the time with my lack of seizure control that we planned to minimise risks to myself and the children in every possible way.

RISK

Minimising risk has to be carefully thought out, and it is something that having experienced myself, I am now able to pass on to my patients with uncontrolled seizures who become parents for the first time. These strategies include such things as advising them to sit on floor cushions whilst feeding their babies in case they have a seizure and fall. This minimises the risk to the mother as well as the child.

Other important examples include changing and dressing the baby on the floor so they cannot fall if the mother has a seizure. Sponging the baby down on a changing mat on the floor is safer than bathing the baby in water. The use of a padded carry-cot will protect the baby if they are dropped, rather than the mother carrying them in her arms.

Other risk management strategies include fitting a deadlock to the pram so that it will stay in one place even if the mother lets go of it. The use of a safety gate may stop a small child or a baby getting to other parts of the home and play-pens may be used to keep young children safe whilst the mother attends to other tasks.

Guards on cookers and fires are also recommended, as is feeding the baby in a short high-chair which is less likely to overbalance than a taller one.

My lack of seizure freedom at this critical time in my children's life was easier to cope with at home than while out and about. It was here that we had the most alarming experiences.

Coping with such a traumatic experience as a parent having a seizure presents a dilemma to the child. It constitutes a role-reversal, even if only a temporary one, where the parent is helpless and to a large extent dependent on the child who becomes the carer. If this is to work, it will be necessary for the child to have learned, preferably by good example, how to cope and what best to do. Although at home we were careful to prepare our children for difficulties that may arise through their mother having a seizure, when out and about we met widespread ignorance concerning what epilepsy meant and how to help. An example of this is that my son was asked "Does mother often do this?" by a customer at the local butcher's shop as he tried to cope with me on the floor on one occasion. It is a fact that members of the public find it very implausible that a small child may cope with this type of situation better than they could themselves. It is not surprising therefore that we often met with a certain amount of hostility including whether I thought it was fair to have had my children at all!

I think it is important to look back on what my children said about our life at that time. In a school essay entitled 'Relatives and how to cope with them', my son wrote:

"My mum has a thing called epilepsy, in other words she has epileptic fits. Every month or so she has them. Although it is hard to see your own mother lying on the ground shaking and dribbling, I have found that, hard as it is, just think how lucky you are it is not you. I know I have a lot of things to worry about but I have learnt how to cope with them so I am not that unlucky."

When I read this I was encouraged to find that as young as my son was he was able to see things in such a comparatively mature way for his age.

My daughter too wrote about the experience of seeing my seizures and described it as quite distressing which I am sure it was, she also described the following:

"Like many young children my brother and I would often play games together. One of our favourite games was playing mummies and daddies. My brother would direct me in my role and I would listen to his instructions.

"This was a great source of amusement to my mother and father who sometimes watched from a distance."

My brother would say "Anna, you're going shopping!" and I would obligingly respond by carrying a shopping bag across the room. I then received my next command, "Now you go to buy some bread". I then pretended to buy a loaf of bread putting my imaginary purse in my bag. This was followed by my brother saying "Now you have a fit!" at which point my shopping trip came to a halt and I fell to the ground and proceeded to act as if I was having a seizure, imitating my mother's convulsions. I did this by making moaning noises combined with making odd movements with my mouth. After this I would lie still until my brother directed me to get up and continue shopping. We often played in this way for quite a while and although this might seem strange, as it is normally not an expected part of the way in which children play, looking back on it now I can see that such role-play was our own way of coming to terms with our mother's condition."

A particularly horrifying experience being a mother with then uncontrolled seizures stands out in mind to this day. I walked to my children's school to collect them each day and on this occasion I must have had a seizure on the way there. A member of the public called for an ambulance and on regaining consciousness in the A & E Department of our local teaching hospital my first thought was for my children. "Where are my children?" I demanded "What children?" came the reply. I managed to impress on them that I had been on my way to collect my children from school, and you can imagine my distress at not knowing whether or not they were safe and where they had got to. It is true to say that anything could have happened but fortunately they traced them eventually thanks to the road safety ('lollipop') lady who was on duty that afternoon at the school. Once all the other children had been met and safely seen across the road she took my children to our home in her car and waited outside the house until I arrived sometime later. I am grateful to her to this day.

ACHIEVING SEIZURE FREEDOM AND LOSING IT

Over the years that I have been seeing patients in my clinic at the hospital for counselling, I have become aware of the immense emotional cost to them when it seems that at last their seizures have come under better control, sometimes for several years, only to relapse again. As a counsellor, what one is dealing with is loss which may be particularly keenly felt at such times. There are all sorts of implications for people in once more losing their seizure freedom which they have treasured.

Looking back over the course of my epilepsy, for many years I had between four and 10 seizures a month. These were severe and often debilitating and it would not be uncommon for me to lose several days of useful life each month after particularly long seizures.

About 11 years ago my seizures increased in frequency and I was eventually admitted to hospital where I had an MRI scan. The lesion responsible for my seizures had bled leading to an exacerbation of my condition as well as several new symptoms such as right-sided weakness and difficulties with speech. Surgery was debated and after further investigations including hours of functional imaging it was decided that I could have the operation.

Following surgery, I had a period of complete freedom from seizures for about 5 months, something which I had never known before. Then one day I had a devastating blow, my first seizure since surgery.

I have to say that even though I am a particularly resilient person used to coping with adversity, I found this experience of suddenly losing the control I had gained quite devastating. It took some time to adjust and during this time I had further seizures.

Thanks to the advent of new anti-epileptic medication which has helped enormously with my seizure control, I now enjoy a better quality of life than I have ever had since my epilepsy was diagnosed. I also suffer far fewer side effects on my current medication in comparison with the older drugs I had to tolerate, which were at the time so debilitating. I have more energy than I ever had when I was younger, and I often describe the relative seizure freedom I have now (about two to three seizures per year) as like living in the Garden of Eden. I never thought that I would be as comparatively well as I am today.

In contrast to some of the patients I see who also enjoy relative freedom from seizures, I am able to appreciate the improvement in my quality of life whole- heartedly. By contrast, I have seen patients for whom this is not the case. The possibility of a seizure is never far from their minds and they live in fear and dread of further attacks. They require a lot of support and it is not uncommon for them to feel very insecure despite the improvements in their seizure control which they fear maybe only temporary.

SOCIAL ISSUES IN RELATION TO SEIZURE FREEDOM

Public perceptions of epilepsy, often shared by patients themselves are evident by the striking array of euphemisms patients and their relatives use to describe the seizures: 'funny turns', 'feeling giddy', 'dizzy spells', 'fainting' and 'blackouts'. Bagley (1971) maintained that there is 'an innate prejudice against epilepsy', rooted in the fear that the sufferer is always liable to sudden, unpredictable and dramatic losses of motor control or to 'going berserk', something 'normal' people fear happening to themselves. Taylor (1969) pointed out that 'the social structure survives through its experience of the value of control, order and reason', and added that 'each seizure reinforces the view that people with epilepsy cannot be relied upon to partic-ipate fully in society, since they are liable, at any time, to go out of control'.

It is then not difficult to see why seizure freedom is so important to both people with epilepsy and society in general. Patients' measure of perceived stigma varies quite a lot but for those in whom it is high, living with uncon-trolled seizures it is all the more difficult and a socially isolating experience. This is sometimes exacerbated by the reaction of the patient's family who frequently harbour fears for their safety and have doubts about their own (the family's that is) ability to cope with the situation. I have known cases where the whole family becomes quite isolated, fearing that a seizure while in company or out and about and may have devastating consequences.

ETHNIC ISSUES

Ethnicity often plays a bit part in the way a diagnosis of epilepsy is perceived. In my clinic I have seen many patients from ethnic minority groups for whom the fact of their epilepsy has been viewed as quite disastrous by their families.

In India, even today, a woman known to have epilepsy has virtually no chance of an arranged marriage. People with epilepsy are often thought to be uneducable, unemployable and a danger to the community. The Yoruba in Nigeria see epilepsy as the sign of a visitation by the devil. Such views are quite widely held in developing countries, but clearly not restricted to them.

Cultural and historical ideas thus influence the opinions of the family and thus the setting in which the person with seizures grows up. It is important to be aware of the enormity of the social stigma that may abound within certain ethnic groups in different parts of the world.

Case Example A

A young woman in her mid 20s was referred to me in my clinic for counselling. She was very unhappy. She told me that, as is the custom in many Asian families she had gone to live with her husband's parents following their marriage. She related to me how whenever the family were expecting guests, she was confined to her bedroom and was not allowed to take part in any social occasion. She clearly felt isolated and depressed at this sad situation and in the course of many conversations with her I learned that neither her husband nor his family were told about her epilepsy prior to the marriage.

She explained to me that this was not uncommon due to the way epilepsy is perceived in India. According to her, if her diagnosis had been known to her in-laws prior to the arranged marriage, marriage for her would have been out of the question. She added, furthermore, that none of her siblings would have been considered marriageable due to the fact that epilepsy is seen as a highly inheritable condition and one which blights any family in which it occurs. She also related that her parents-in-law seldom spoke to her, such was their fear and shame.

Although this seems a very extreme example to the western mind, I understand that it is the norm in many parts of the Asian sub-continent.

Case Example B

A young woman aged about 30 was referred to me as being in need of support. She was the mother of two-year-old twin sons and was finding it difficult to cope. She was of Arabian Middle Eastern origin and was living in the UK. She explained that she had been diagnosed with seizures about 18 months before when her baby sons were about six months old. She went on to tell me that as soon as she was diagnosed, her husband had left her and she had to cope alone with the boys. He was now living elsewhere although he did attend her hospital follow-up appointments with her.

She was extremely distressed and at the same time understandably anxious about how her boys would be affected by both the departure of their father and her uncontrolled seizures when he was not around to ensure her safety and that of his sons. She explained to me that the community in their country of origin viewed epilepsy as highly undesirable and stigmatising and she felt this had influenced her husband in his decision to leave. She added that in her opinion, the reason why her husband attended her hospital appointments with her was merely to make it appear that he had not left the marital home and was still living there.

Case Example C

A young University graduate, whose parents had come to this country before his birth, was referred to me by his neurologist as being in need of support and counselling. It emerged that he was having employment problems and had been moved by the company where he worked to another department when he had had a seizure at work. He had never made a secret of his seizures and worked in the accounts department. He had been relocated to a position which he was very unhappy about.

Over the months that I saw this patient for regular sessions, I discovered that this was merely the tip of the iceberg in terms of the unhappiness he suffered. It turned out that whenever he called home from London to Birmingham to speak to his parents, or younger sister, his father would answer the telephone and on recognising his son's voice, would immediately hang up. This poor young man received no support from his family and, although he had been born in the UK and gone to school and University here, his parents still clung to the beliefs of the community in which they had been brought up in Asia.

He felt he had nowhere to turn for support and was being victimised both by his family and work colleagues. The contact he had with me over the many months that I saw him, became very important.

The three case examples which I have given are not uncommon amongst ethnic groups and it is important to realise just how threatening a condition epilepsy in its refractory form is seen to be.

LABELLING

The tendency to have uncontrolled seizures frequently attracts labelling. The patients I see bitterly complain about being labelled by their family, friends and colleagues as 'epileptic'. On occasion, they even use this term to describe themselves but most prefer to use the term 'a person with epilepsy'. There is a move towards some people disliking the term 'patient', feeling that this implies passivity and lack of control. They resent the image these terms imply and the stigma which surrounds their condition.

It is difficult to say exactly how long such labelling may endure following seizure freedom. In the case of social services, the receipt of benefits may cease after the patient has been rendered seizure-free for a year.

When considering epilepsy surgery it is important that the patient and their family be made aware of this and the possible responsibility they would face if their operation were to be completely successful. In such cases, the time would come when they would no longer be considered disabled and therefore would not qualify for the benefits they had been receiving in the past. It is important to have a plan that goes beyond seizure freedom and takes into account what happens next.

A further difficulty with labelling may be the label that patients give to themselves. This may have a profound psychological affect on them and their own self-perception.

I have often found in my clinical practice that patients who consider themselves disabled also have a set of sometimes quite unshakable beliefs surrounding disability that maybe difficult for them and others to deal with. I consider myself fortunate in that I have never considered myself disabled and therefore any labelling that others might attach to me has gone largely over my head.

The great majority of people referred to me for counselling hold the opposite view. On the one hand they deeply resent the labelling they believe that people attach to them and on the other they use these labels to describe themselves and the things that happen to them.

It is very common in my view for people to believe that their social prospects are virtually nil because people will see them as 'epileptic'. I explain to them that in fact their seizures may be epileptic (used as an adjective) but that does not make them an 'epileptic' (noun). I see epilepsy as only one aspect of a person's life, a detail of their medical history rather than a defining term. I encourage people to see themselves in a more rounded way and not just in terms of their medical diagnosis. I often ask them what other terms they might use to describe themselves other than 'epileptic' or 'disabled'. It is true that some people struggle to find other terms they feel readily apply to them, but with patience and encouragement they do generally eventually achieve this.

SELF ESTEEM

There are of course many factors that make up a person's self esteem but certainly their perceived quality of life is an important one and is something that varies enormously within a group of people with uncontrolled seizures. Those who feel continually tired and fatigued as well as those who complain of memory and concentration difficulties already have a constant drain on their resources. This often results in them feeling lonely and isolated and may influence their ability to attract a partner or even have any sort of social life let alone a sexual relationship.

Stigma and self esteem

With increasing political correctness has come a real awareness of stereotyping by means of language. I have noted a very acute sensitivity in many people with seizures at being called 'epileptic'. While it is commonplace to refer to people with diabetes as 'diabetic' and those with asthma as 'asthmatic' there is a feeling amongst people with epilepsy that the term 'epileptic' in itself is prejudicial. Their perception of the term is a negative one as is the language which encapsulates it. There are many schools of thought about this particular phenomenon, for example in American medical schools the term 'epileptic' is discouraged because it is thought to be derogatory. The feeling seems to be also that the term 'fits' is offensive and it is not any longer used by medical personnel. I can understand that it is easy for a medical student to be taught 'known epileptic' as an easy way of writing off someone with epilepsy.

It is interesting to note how this type of labelling varies from disease to disease. Other long-term neurological conditions for example Parkinson's disease or Multiple Sclerosis are associated in the public mind with famous people who have had them. They have been quite open about the fact that they have the disease and helped to raise money and the profile of the illness. In the case of epilepsy this has not happened, and begs the question as to how far stereotyping and labelling is seen as negative in people with seizures. The net effect of this is often that people with epilepsy themselves are perpetuating the closet nature of the condition and I find this rather sad.

LIBIDO AND EPILEPSY

Sexual dysfunction, notably hypo-sexuality is often reported to me by patients I see in the clinic. This particular problem seems to be greatest in those with temporal lobe epilepsy. Some studies show that the incidence of hypo-sexuality is twice as high in these patients as in those with primary generalised seizures.

Hypo-sexuality, or low libido, may continue to be reported regardless of the degree of seizure control the patient has. Women on the whole seem to find it less difficult to talk about their hypo-sexuality than do men who are very sensitive to the term impotence. Both epilepsy and impotence are often felt by men to be equally stigmatising and it may take many years before they are able to admit to having potency problems to anyone.

Some recent studies show that the rate of impotency in men with epilepsy maybe as high as in diabetes. If this is so, there maybe an argument for the prescribing of such medications as Viagra on the NHS for them.

I sometimes see adolescent women in clinic who fear sexual activity believing that a seizure during intercourse may spoil their partner's feelings for them. Concern about the possibility of a seizure occurring during sexual activity is not uncommon in women with uncontrolled seizures and they sometimes report in some ways fearing being out of control during sexual intercourse and equating this with the loss of control attached to their seizures.

I have seen both male and female patients in my clinic reporting that they have no sex drive whatsoever. To date there are very few recommendations or guidelines for this type of difficulty and yet it is responsible for a lot of emotional turmoil and difficulties within relationships.

CONCLUSION

There can be little doubt about the improvement in medical and surgical treatments of epilepsy during recent years. Minimising or abolishing seizures will always be the aim of both clinician and patient alike and I hope this chapter has helped to set out some of the reasons for this. Although there may potentially be some difficulties in achieving seizure freedom for a minority of patients, appropriate help and support may assist them with adjusting to this new way of living and its potential advantages.

I am pleased to have been asked to write about this subject from the patient's view point and to have had the chance to include my own experiences with poorly controlled epilepsy over many years. I hope this has illustrated just how much the recent advances in treatment have helped to minimise the risk of mortality, morbidity, psychological and emotional difficulties in people with epilepsy. It is my personal hope that seizure freedom will be a realistic possibility for an increasing number of people diagnosed with seizures in the years to come.

Acknowledgements

I thank Andrew, Oliver and Anna Usiskin for their encouragement over many years. I also thank Professor Trimble for the opportunity to contribute to this book and Jill Rayfield for her help with typing my manuscript.

REFERENCES

Bagley, C. (1971) *The Social Psychology of the Child with Epilepsy*. Routledge & Kegan Paul, London, p113.

Shorvon, S.D. and Farmer, P.J. (1989) Epilepsy in Developing Countries. In: Trimble, M.R. (Ed), *Chronic Epilepsy, its Prognosis and Management*. John Wiley & Sons, Chichester, pp 223-224.

Taylor, D. (1969) Some Psychiatric Aspects of Epilepsy. In: Herrington, R. (Ed), *Current Problems in Neuropsychiatry*. Healey, Ashford, p.107.

Seizure Freedom: Clinical, Research and Quality of Life Perspectives
Edited by Michael R. Trimble
© 2006 Clarius Press Ltd

10

Seizures, Seizure Freedom
and Cognition

CARL B. DODRILL

*Departments of Neurology, Neurological Surgery, and Psychiatry,
University of Washington School of Medicine,
Seattle, Washington, USA*

INTRODUCTION

This chapter deals with two related questions:

1) the impacts of seizures upon cognition, and,

2) the impacts of the absence of seizures upon cognition once the seizures have become established.

As will be seen, the answers to these two questions are not necessarily the same.

Regarding the first question, the possibility that seizures may damage the brain and therefore reduce cognitive functioning has been considered for decades. However, the question is an extraordinarily complex one, and the answers to it are still being debated. Only a few years ago, a week long symposium of the world's experts was organised to address this question, and the resulting monograph (Sutula and Pitkanen, 2002) shows how complicated the question actually is. Among other factors, the critical variables to be considered in responding to the question include whether animals or humans are being assessed, the types of seizure under consideration, and the temporal patterns of seizures. Unfortunately, the results are not as clear as we would like them to be.

The possibility that freedom from seizures may have a favourable impact upon cognition is of interest from every perspective. For example, neuropsychological studies of people with epilepsy routinely show that, taken as a whole, performances on a variety of cognitive tasks are at least slightly diminished, and, with difficult to manage groups of seizure patients, are often substantially worse than average. If we could rid them of seizures, perhaps there would be an improvement in cognitive function, with the potential for improvement in cognition of potentially millions of people. Improved cognitive functioning provides the possibility for improvement in daily life performance, and if this could be achieved, the results would be striking indeed. In addition, quality of life changes (see also Chapter 12 of this book) and other favourable alterations accompanying seizure-freedom would certainly have a synergistic effect with the final product being a favourable one indeed. Unfortunately, there are just as many complicating factors in the study of the effects of cessation of seizures as the effects of seizures themselves, with the result that the conclusions drawn cannot as firm as any of us would wish.

Despite the vagaries of the information bearing on both questions, let us consider them in turn in the light of selective literature reviews and see if some general conclusions cannot be reasonably drawn.

THE EFFECTS OF SEIZURES UPON COGNITION

There has been a tremendous amount written about this topic, but the same conclusions have frequently not been drawn, and they have not always been based upon firm empirical groundings. In an effort to resolve at least some of these difficulties, the current review is selective in nature, and it includes only studies which had the following features:

1) formal tests of mental abilities were used rather than clinical judgments of cognitive functioning; and

2) patients with epilepsy were tested on at least two occasions without an intervening treatment such as surgery or systematic drug changes which may have impacted the test results.

Thus, it was insisted that the data upon which conclusions would be drawn should be as reliable as possible. Also, since cross-sectional studies can be contaminated by coexisting variables, it was required that all studies reviewed here were longitudinal investigations. Longitudinal studies are likely to present the most accurate information as cross-sectional studies attribute more adverse cognitive changes to seizures than can be documented by longitudinal investigations (Dodrill, 2002). Taking these two requirements together, in order for a study to be included in the review, formal testing must have been accomplished at both the beginning and the end of a study. Studies meeting these requirements will be reviewed first for children and then for adults.

Studies involving children

Table 1 summarises the results of the nine longitudinal studies done with children that could be found. Of immediate interest is the fact that there are no fewer than five of these investigations done before 1940. Clearly, this has been a topic of interest for decades, and as will become apparent, there was earlier interest in this with children than with adults. Also readily evident from Table 1 is the fact that the outcome measures were routinely indicators of intelligence and intelligence only. Indeed, every study used either one form or another of the Binet or the Wechsler intelligence scales. Unfortunately, this is a limitation of this group of investigations because measures of intelligence are not as sensitive to difficulties in brain functions as are validated neuropsychological tests (Reitan and Wolfson, 1993). Measures of intelligence were, after all, not devised to identify brain-related problems but to predict how well children would do in school (Matarazzo, 1972). The neuropsychological tests used today clearly evaluate a broader range of functions than do measures of intelligence.

An additional and unfortunate limitation is also obvious from Table 1, and this is that there are very few data presented on frequency of seizures between the testings. As best as can be determined, all children had active seizure disorders except for those in a single investigation (Ellenberg *et al.*, 1986). Of the eight remaining reports, there was evidence for some cognitive loss in every investigation except for one (Patterson and Fonner, 1928). In fact, IQ losses of 10 points or more were commonly reported in about 10-25% of the children studied. The data on seizure type and seizure frequency are so sparse that no clear connections between these variables and adverse cognitive changes can be made. Nevertheless, the weight of the evidence is that measurable losses in intelligence were experienced over time in at least a portion of the children with active seizures. Furthermore, these studies all had test-retest intervals of only 1-4 years. Longer intervals would likely have resulted in more findings.

Studies involving adolescents and adults

A total of 13 longitudinal investigations with adolescents and adults were found, and their summary results are presented in Table 2. Only five of the 13 studies rested on measures of intelligence alone, and in general, the results relied upon data that were more diverse by nature than was the case with children. Also, three of the studies evaluated cognitive changes over 10 year periods, on average, and thus the test-retest periods were distinctively longer. Nevertheless, the seizure type and seizure frequency information were often no more precisely given than with children, although admittedly there were a few exceptions where these data were more clearly reported (Dodrill, 2002; Dodrill and Wilensky, 1990; Holmes *et al.*, 1998; Selwa *et al.*, 1994).

In two studies in Table 2 (Dodrill and Wilensky, 1992; Aikia and Kalviainen, 1999), patients had few or no seizures between testings, and in these cases test performances either remained the same or improved. In the remaining 11 investigations, one can assume that most patients had at least a few seizures during the study period even though it was rarely possible to specify even approximately how many seizures had actually been experienced. Among the 11, evidence was found for a relationship between seizures and adverse cognitive changes in five (Dodrill and Wilensky, 1990; Helmstaedter et al., 2003; Holmes et al., 1998; Rodin, 1968; Seidenberg et al., 1981), mixed or uncertain findings in four (Arief and Yacorzynski, 1942; Helmstaedter et al., 2000; Helmstaedter et al., 2003), and no connection between seizures and cognitive change was found in two instances (Bjornaes et al., 2001; Selwa et al., 1994). These findings must be described as mixed when considered as a whole. However, an examination of the last column in Table 2 reveals a series of observations, all of which would support a mild connection between seizures and adverse cognitive change. These findings include statistically significant correlations between numbers of seizures (or presence of intervening status epilepticus) and decreased scores on tests of abilities (Dodrill, 2002; Dodrill and Wilensky, 1990; Rodin, 1968), changes in intelligence corresponding to changes in seizure frequency (Seidenberg et al., 1981), better performances over time with normals than with people with epilepsy (Dodrill, 2002), and losses in mental abilities with patients having uncontrolled seizures which touch on a number of areas of cognitive functioning (Holmes et al., 1998) even though it is commonly believed that losses in memory are the most frequent (Dodrill, 2002; Helmstaedter et al., 2000; Helmstaedter et al., 2003).

In summary, for the first basic question addressed in this chapter relative to adverse changes in cognition, it is concluded that losses in mental abilities do occur over time with uncontrolled seizures in patients with epilepsy. Such changes may be more easily found in children than in adults, as was demonstrated in the review as a whole. The impression gained by the author of this chapter is that losses in mental abilities are most easily connected with generalised tonic-clonic seizures, especially when experienced in a serial fashion (status epilepticus) and without warning (more likely to result and falls and head injuries). However, it is also the belief of this author that even single isolated convulsive seizures are likely to be associated with diminished mental abilities if enough are allowed to accumulate, such as more than 100 in total. At the present time it is not possible to make such a statement regarding partial seizures.

Table 1. Longitudinal cognitive studies of children with epilepsy.

Investigator(s)/year	Subject group(s)	Test(s) used	Test-retest interval	Seizure frequency	Cognitive Outcome
Fox (1924)	130 institutionalised children with epilepsy	Binet	One year	Unclear; probably active seizures	37%-decrease>2 IQ points 41%-same-IQ (+/- 2 points) 22%-increase>2 IQ points 8%-decrease>10 IQ points
Patterson and Fonner (1928)	98 institutionalised children and adolescents	Stanford-Binet	12-46 months	Unclear; probably active seizures	34%-decrease>2 IQ points 31%-same-IQ +/- 2 points 34%-increase>2 IQ points
Dawson and Conn (1929)	21 children with epilepsy	Binet	8-56 months	Not stated	Mean IQ drop from 82 to 67; 11 showed losses, 10 no change
Fetterman and Barnes (1934)	46 hospital dispensary cases	Stanford-Binet	21 months on average	Not stated	50%-'moderate loss'; 9% no change; 41%-'slight increase'
Sullivan & Gahagan (1935)	44 children 7.5 years of age; outpatients	Stanford-Binet	1-59 months; 14 months average	Not well described	50%-'negative change'; 5%-'no change'; 45%-'positive Change'; 9%-clear deterioration
Bourgeois et al. (1983)	72 children 7.5 years of age; outpatients	Age-appropriate IQ and other tests	4 years on average	Details provided at length; active seizure disorders	No change in IQ for the group overall, but IQ>10 point loss in 11% who had frequent seizures, toxic drug levels, early epilepsy
Ellenberg, et al. (1986)	83 children from a large Developmental study	Stanford-Binet at age 4; WISC at age 7	3 years	Patients had very few seizures	Intelligence showed no losses from age 3 to age 7
Aldenkamp et al. (1990)	45 children 9.3 years of age; outpatients	Dutch form of the WISC-R	4.2 years on average	All but 10 children had active seizures through follow-up	IQ scores slightly but not significantly down for total group; 24% had FSIQ losses>9 points
Bjornaes et al. (2001)	17 children 10.2 years of age; later had surgery	Norwegian form of the WISC-R	3.5 years on average	All had active seizures of moderate severity	Adverse IQ score changes found PIQ (p<.05), FSIQ (p<.05)

Table 2.   Longitudinal cognitive studies of adolescents and adults with epilepsy.

Investigator(s)/year	Subject group(s)	Test(s) used	Test-retest interval	Seizure frequency	Cognitive Outcome
Arieff and Yacorzynski (1942)	90 adolescents and adults; 27 known etiology, 63 unknown etiology	Binet, 1916 and 1937 versions	1 to 10 years	Wide range of seizure control from complete remission to very active	Significant loss of 6 IQ points if aetiology was known; no loss when aetiology was unknown
Rodin (1968)	56 adolescents and adults	Wechsler-Bellevue, Form I (?)	At least 5 years, 7 years on average	Wide range of seizure control	Favourable changes in seizure frequency correlated .33 (p<.02) with favourable changes in FSIQ
Seidenberg et al. (1981)	47 adults; 22 improved in seizure frequency; 25 had no change or got worse	WAIS	1-5 years, 18 months on average	Varied by subgroup	Seizure improved group had 3-10 IQ point improvements; seizure unimproved group had −1 to +4 point changes
Dodrill and Wilensky (1990)	9 adults with status epilepticus during the study period, and 9 closely matched controls with no history of status	WAIS	5 years (+/- 6 months)	One group with status (4 GTC, 5 partial), one the group without status	The no status group improved more on FSIQ than did status group (p<.05); same trend shown on VIQ
Kalska (1991)	69 adults who had participated in a vocational rehabilitation program	Finnish form of the WAIS; tests of memory and some other functions	Approximately 10 years	Improved in control over study, but only 10% controlled at end	Memory losses in 15-20%; intelligence unchanged overall; seizure frequency and losses in abilities difficult to connect
Dodrill and Wilensky (1992)	36 adults with no medication changes over a 5 year period	Expanded Halstead-Reitan battery, WAIS	5 years (+/- 6 months)	Very few or no seizures	No changes on the tests beyond those expected by chance
Selwa et al. (1994)	28 adults with TLE, typically with complaints of memory problems	WAIS-R, Wechsler Memory Scale (Form I)	2.3 years on average	8 partial seizures per month	Slight improvement in PIQ and FSIQ as would be expected by chance in a normal adult group

Table 2 continued on next page

Table 2. (*Continued*) Longitudinal cognitive studies of adolescents and adults with epilepsy.

Investigator(s)/year	Subject group(s)	Test(s) used	Test-retest interval	Seizure frequency	Cognitive Outcome
Holmes *et al.* (1998)	35 adults with intractable partial seizures (60% also had secondary GTC)	Expanded Halstead-Reitan battery, WAIS	10 years (+/- 6 months)	9 partial and general-ised seizures per month	WAIS little change; 6/17 other test variables showed losses (visual memory, attention, problem solving, perception)
Aikia and Kalviainen (1999)	58 new cases with partial seizures	Finnish form of the WAIS and other tests	5 years	Very few seizures of any kind	12/24 test variables showed slight gains; none showed losses
Helmstaedter *et al.* (2000)	47 TLE cases	Measures of memory and other functions	2-10 years, 4.7 years on average	Active partial seizures especially	Verbal memory unchanged; figural memory showed a loss (p<.05)
Bjornaes *et al.* (2001)	17 adults who became surgical candidates	WAIS	6 years	Mild to moderate seizure severity (mean of 2.3 on a 0-4 scale)	No losses found. Better PIQ (p<.01) and FSIQ (p<.05) may have been retest effects
Dodrill (2002)	35 adults with partial seizures with or without secondary generalization; 35 normal controls	Expanded Halstead-Reitan battery, WAIS	10 years (+/- 6 months)	Average of 1,109 partial seizure and 61 GTC over 10 years for epilepsy group. Four patients experienced GTC status epilepticus during the 10 year period	Normal group improved more than epilepsy group on 3/20 test variables. Visual memory lost in both groups. Partial seizures not correlated with ability changes, but 2/20 significantly correlated with number of GTCs. GTC status patients lost verbal and visual memory
Helmstaedter *et al.* (2003)	102 adults with TLE	Measures of memory and of some other cognitive functions	2 to 10 years, average of 57 months	89% had more than 1/month at start, 72% had more than 1/month at end of study	50% showed significant decline in memory (verbal plus figural combined); few changes in non-memory functions

COGNITIVE CORRELATES OF FREEDOM FROM SEIZURES

If adverse cognitive change with repeated seizures can be shown over time, can improved cognitive functioning be found to be related to cessation of seizures? While this area is a potentially promising one, it also raises cautions about approaching the problem in a manner which is too simple minded with the danger of drawing conclusions that do not recognise the complexities of the situation. Both the literature will be reviewed on the topic and new data will also be presented in an effort to cast as much light as possible on this area.

Surgery for epilepsy—literature review

The best place to begin is likely with regard to surgery for epilepsy, for this is the one intervention which is most likely to make a dramatic alteration in seizure frequency and in fact to make a person seizure-free. A review of the literature was therefore undertaken, but it was quickly discovered that, whereas many studies have been published on cognitive changes (especially memory) after epilepsy surgery, it is much less frequent that such changes are reported in relation to extent of seizure relief. More frequently, cognitive changes after epilepsy surgery are commonly studied in a predictive context or in a context that pertains to relating them to the type of surgery performed. Nevertheless, several investigations were found which explicitly did related cognitive changes following epilepsy surgery to changes in seizure frequency, and they are summarised in Table 3.

In order to evaluate adequately the cognitive change after epilepsy surgery, a review of the findings in Table 3 must take into account whether surgery was on the same side as cerebral dominance for speech. As is well known, surgery on the speech (usually left) side is frequently associated with adverse changes in mental abilities, especially verbal memory. Also, whether or not mesial temporal sclerosis is present is related to cognitive change after surgery, with a greater adverse change likely when mesial temporal sclerosis is not present, so that healthy tissue was likely removed at the time of surgery. The simultaneous appearance of both of these findings is noted in Seidenberg *et al.* (1998). Here, the mesial temporal sclerosis groups did not show any change, good or bad, and this was true even though there was substantial relief from seizures in the typical case. Also, the right non-mesial temporal sclerosis group did not lose mental abilities after surgery, but the left group did lose verbal abilities with such losses being unrelated to relief from seizures. Thus, the side of surgery and the presence vs. absence of mesial temporal sclerosis bore a stronger relationship to cognitive change than did relief from seizures.

A review of the remaining studies summarised in Table 3 reveals very mixed findings. About half the time, a mild relationship between cognitive status after surgery and relief from seizures was reported, always in the

Table 3. Studies reporting results on cognitive changes in relationship to relief from seizures following epilepsy surgery.

Author(s) and date	Patients group(s) studied	Sub-groups	Outcome: Cognitive changes after epilepsy surgery
Lieb et al. (1982)	36 adults with TLE; 7.6 year average follow-up	None—patients analyzed as a group	Changes in WAIS IQ scores (pre-post) were significantly negatively correlated with relief from seizures after surgery (VIQ -.57, p<.001; PIQ -.37, p<.05; FSIQ .60 p<.001) but not with WMS MQ (r= -.18)
Novelly et al., (1984)	23 adults receiving anterior temporal lobectomies; 12 month follow-up period	Side of surgery: speech-side (n=10) vs. other side (n=13). Seizure relief: good (n=18) vs. poor (n=5)	IQ and memory scores improved with good seizure relief but tended not to change with poor relief or to be slightly worse. IQ scores improved more when surgery was on the side opposite speech than when it was on the speech side
Seidenberg et al. (1998)	Non-retarded adults with typical speech representation plus a control group of nonsurgical epilepsy patient controls	LTL surgery (n=54); RTL surgery (n=34); each group divided into mesial sclerosis present vs. absent; 40 controls	MTS groups did not show cognitive change; the LTL non-MTS group lost verbal memory, naming, and verbal conceptual abilities, but these losses were unrelated to seizure relief. Perceptual organization factor slightly worse if not seizure-free after surgery
Martin et al. (2000)	Nonretarded adults with typical speech representation; 7 month follow-up on average	LTL surgery (n=94); RTL surgery (n=80); amygdale and anterior 2/3 of hippocampus taken	Patients who were seizure-free (71% of all cases) had significantly improved (p <.001) verbal fluency (COWAT) over patients who were not seizure-free but showed no difference in concept formation (WCST) or problem solving (Trail Making, Part B)
Rausch et al. (2003)	Nonretarded adults without gross structural lesions; speech always on left; 9-19 year follow-up	LTL surgery (n=21); RTL surgery (n=23); anterior 2 cm of hippocampus and 2/3 of amygdala removed	Little relationship found between relief from seizures and cognitive change at either 1 year or 12 years after surgery, although 77% of the sample was seizure-free at long-term (12 year) follow-up

Table 3 continued on next page

Table 3. (Continued) Studies reporting results on cognitive changes in relationship to relief from seizures following epilepsy surgery.

Author(s) and date	Patients group(s) studied	Sub-groups	Outcome: Cognitive changes after epilepsy surgery
Suchy et al. (2003)	Nonretarded adults with typical speech representation; frontal and temporal cases included; 7 months average follow-up period	LTL surgery (n=81); RTL surgery (n=71); LFL surgery (n=8); RFL surgery (n=14)	Verbal and nonverbal fluency generally lower if seizures continued after surgery; no impact of type of fluency, side of surgery, or site of surgery (frontal vs. temporal)
Baxendale & Thompson (2005)	Broad range of cases with preoperative and one-year postoperative evaluations; all had ATL surgeries	LTL surgery (n=157); RTL surgery (n=133)	Seizure-free and not seizure-free patients did not differ in degree of change in verbal memory after surgery
Sanyal et al. (2005)	Nonretarded, right handed adults without contralateral pathology; 8 month average follow-up	LTL surgery (n=12); LTL surgery (n=13)	No change in cognition with LTL patients, regardless of degree of relief from seizures. In RTL patients, no relief from seizures was associated with no cognitive change, but good relief from seizures (Engel I & II) was associated with improvement in memory and in intelligence

expected direction but with different forms of it being expressed. With freedom from seizures, sometimes there was actual improvement in cognition, but at other times the seizure-free person just did not get worse (as did the people with continued attacks), but with almost half the studies showing no real cognitive changes at all, even with the substantial relief from seizures which was typically experienced. It was concluded that in a surgical context, there may be a slightly favorable cognitive result with people who have been rendered seizure-free by epilepsy surgery as to those who have not. Measures of especially verbal fluency are perhaps most likely to show this change, but any such change is likely to be limited in degree and it is to be found only a portion of the time.

The findings just summarised must be rectified with the common report of patients after surgeries that they are better cognitively than they were before the surgery, and especially better in the area of memory. There are now at least three papers that deal specifically with this issue among patients who have had surgery for their seizures (Cañizares *et al.*, 2000; Lineweaver *et al.*, 2004; McGlone, 1994). These papers are unanimous in suggesting that factors other than actual memory are responsible for the self-reported cognitive change. Patients are likely to confuse improvement in seizures with improved memory. In addition, emotional disturbance of a neurotic nature can have a decided impact upon reports of memory and memory change. The importance of emotional factors in patient self-evaluation of memory has also been confirmed in a number of other groups of people including patients who have had cardiac surgery (Vingerhoets, 1998), chronic fatigue syndrome (Vercoulen *et al.*, 1998), head injuries (Gass and Apple, 1997), and in war veterans (Binder *et al.*, 1999).

Surgery for epilepsy—original study

The results from the studies cited above regarding cognitive change following epilepsy surgery are less than ideal for several reasons. For one thing, the literature review did not truly answer the question of whether there are or are not cognitive changes after successful surgery for epilepsy. Irregular periods of follow-up within most studies is another issue in part because it suggests that follow-ups were obtained on a 'catch as catch can' basis, with the length of the follow-up period varying significantly from one patient to the next within most studies. While variable intervals from surgery to cognitive testing are of concern in and of themselves, follow-ups done on that basis may well have a bias towards including people referred for repeat testing because they were not doing especially well after surgery. The scope of the batteries of tests given was often limited by practical considerations, especially at follow-up where available time is often limited. Finally, in order to firmly connect changes in cognitive status with changes in seizure frequency, it would appear important to have enough subjects so that analyses could be conducted by various ranges of seizure relief after surgery, and more than just 'seizure-free' or 'not seizure-free'. In order to deal with these concerns, and in an effort to provide more definitive information on the topic central to this paper, an original investigation was undertaken, and this is described below.

Several years ago the author led a study of the cognitive changes after surgery, the results of which have never been reported in relationship to relief from seizures. Colleagues on this study were Linda M. Ojemann, Lawrence Batzel, Nancy Temkin, and Robert Fraser, to whom the present writer is greatly indebted. Patients were identified who had undergone cortical resection surgery for epilepsy in any cortical area five years previously (+/- 6 months) or 10 years previously (+/- 6 months). Each patient must have had surgery at our centre and a complete neuropsychological evaluation prior to surgery. Each must also have been reachable and willing to come in for a two-day evaluation. This evaluation included a neurological examination, waking and sleeping EEGs, and a complete neuropsychological assessment. Strenuous efforts were made to obtain every qualifying patient for this study, the patients were compensated for their time, and their expenses were paid. There were 74 people in the 5-year group and 34 people in the 10-year group who met all of these qualifications and who actually completed the study.

Taken together, the groups averaged 26.2 (SD = 7.2) years of age at the onset of the study, and an average of 33.7 (SD = 7.3) years of age at the end of the study. They averaged 12.3 (SD = 2.7) years of education at the start of the study. There were 53 men and 55 women. All but one was Caucasian. The right hand was used for writing in 94 cases and the left hand in 14. Average at onset of repetitive seizures was 10.5 years (SD = 6.0), and the average number of seizures experienced per month in the two years prior to surgery was 7.8 (SD = 9.3). On none of these variables did the 5-year follow-up group and the 10-year follow-up groups differ prior to surgery. Before surgery and at follow-up, each patient was administered the complete Wechsler Adult Intelligence Scale (WAIS) and the Neuropsychological Battery for Epilepsy which is an expanded Halstead-Reitan battery (Dodrill, 1978).

Relief from seizures was categorised as follows:

1) *Seizure-free*—No seizures at all in the last two years of follow-up but auras were permitted;
2) *Significantly Improved*—At least a 75% improvement in seizure frequently in the last two years of follow-up compared to the last two years before surgery; and,
3) *Not Significantly Improved*—Less than a 75% improvement in the last two years of follow-up.

There were 53 (49%) people in the Seizure-free Group, 30 (28%) in the Significantly Improved Group, and 25 (23%) in the Not Significantly Improved Group. Application of one way repeated measures analysis of various across these groups to the cognitive data resulted in the findings presented in Table 4.

In Table 4, the main effect 'Over time' gives an index as to whether or not there was general improvement on the test variable across patients from before surgery to after surgery. Although not an entirely pure measure, this can be viewed an index of practice or retest effects. As can be seen, the intellectual measures had a considerable degree of practice effect shown, and especially so on those of visual-spatial functioning. This, of course, is well known. The neuropsychological measures did not have as many of these effects.

The main effect 'Across seizure relief groups' identifies those variables where there was a difference in level of performance across the groups that existed pre- and post-surgically that was not attributable to the surgery itself. Again, such effects were found more consistently on the intellectual than on the neuropsychological measures. It is of interest that a patient had a greater chance of becoming seizure-free with a higher preoperative Full Scale IQ. Likewise, the less patients were impaired on the neuropsychological test battery, the more likely that they would be seizure-free after surgery. Speed of simple reading (Stroop Test, reading words), writing (Name Writing), finger tapping (Finger Tapping Test), simple attention/problem solving (Trail Making, Part A), more complex attention/problem solving (Trail Making, Part B), and attention (Rhythm) all showed differences across the seizure relief groups even at the beginning of the study. This finding is of interest in its own right. Further, a review of the data across the seizure relief groups shows that the greatest distinction here was between people who did and who did not become seizure-free at long-term follow-up.

The 'Time by group interaction' effect is of the greatest interest as it evaluates the cognitive changes following surgery that are directly related to the degree of seizure relief following surgery. The IQ scores and a number of the neuropsychological measures showed statistically significant changes that always pointed to greater improvement in test scores with greater relief from seizures. For example, on average, on the WAIS Full Scale IQ score, persons who were Seizure-free gained approximately eight IQ points, people who were Significantly Improved gained approximately five IQ points, and persons who were Not Significantly Improved lost about half of one point. Likewise, on the summary measure from the 16 neuropsychological tests, persons who became Seizure-free had an average of 12% fewer tests outside normal limits at follow-up, those who were Significantly Improved had an average of 1% fewer tests outside normal limits, and those who were Not Significantly Improved were outside normal limits on 4% more of tests at follow-up than they were pre-surgically.

The underlying F statistics are of interest in Table 4 as they provide additional insights. The larger the F statistic, the greater the statistical effect,

Table 4.   A comparison of pre-operative vs. post-operative performances on the WAIS and on selected variables of the Neuropsychological Battery for Epilepsy across seizure relief groups.

Test variable		Before surgery		At 5/10 yr. follow-up		Statistical significance		
		M	SD	M	SD	Over time	Across seizure relief groups	Time x group interaction
WAIS								
Verbal IQ	SF	96.64	14.67	101.43	15.15	.005 F = 8.15	.026 F = 3.78	.001 F = 15.48
	SI	93.73	13.06	97.07	13.80			
	NSI	91.48	12.21	88.44	12.73			
Performance IQ	SF	95.25	12.99	91.10	13.73	.001 F = 67.41	.001 F = 7.48	.001 F = 7.47
	SI	91.10	13.73	98.03	18.38			
	NSI	86.40	10.87	89.40	12.32			
Full Scale IQ	SF	95.50	13.78	103.12	15.14	.001 F = 44.62	.003 F = 6.20	.001 F = 15.22
	SI	91.90	11.32	97.23	14.09			
	NSI	88.52	11.12	87.96	11.74			
Neuropsychological Battery for Epilepsy								
*Stroop Test, reading words (seconds)	SF	102.40	28.26	89.25	22.33	n.s. F = 0.29	.001 F = 9.00	.001 F = 11.00
	SI	123.67	54.82	116.23	48.77			
	NSI	116.57	26.50	142.87	58.53			
Stroop Test, interference (seconds)	SF	264.79	89.24	214.44	77.31	.035 F = 4.58	.017 F = 4.24	.001 F = 10.50
	SI	296.47	127.26	273.23	114.18			
	NSI	283.43	62.19	311.61	111.16			
*Stroop Test, interference minus reading words (seconds)	SF	157.44	59.04	124.44	60.42	n.s. F = 2.63	n.s. F = 2.25	.008 F = 5.10
	SI	166.53	70.70	156.77	76.19			
	NSI	164.78	54.47	177.87	102.19			
*WMS (I) Verbal memory, immediate	SF	17.40	7.31	16.91	6.32	.006 F = 7.95	n.s. F = 0.90	.049 F = 3.10
	SI	18.50	5.34	17.70	6.89			
	NSI	18.13	6.75	13.75	7.66			
WMS (I) Verbal memory, delayed	SF	13.37	7.54	14.16	6.80	n.s. F = 2.74	n.s. F = 0.96	.004 F = 5.93
	SI	13.18	6.94	13.71	7.93			
	NSI	13.91	7.59	9.05	7.74			
*WMS (I) Visual memory, immediate	SF	8.75	2.81	9.00	2.95	n.s. F = 3.06	n.s. F = 0.38	n.s. F = 2.50
	SI	8.67	3.19	8.17	3.01			
	NSI	8.96	2.99	7.83	3.69			

Table 4. (*continued*) A comparison of pre-operative vs. post-operative performances on the WAIS and on selected variables of the Neuropsychological Battery for Epilepsy across seizure relief groups.

Test variable		Before surgery		At 5/10 yr. follow-up		Statistical significance		
		M	SD	M	SD	Over time	Across seizure relief groups	Time x group interaction
WMS (I) Visual memory, delayed	SF	7.15	3.62	7.54	2.93	n.s. F = 3.76	n.s. F = 1.20	.033 F = 3.56
	SI	7.12	3.81	6.46	4.41			
	NSI	6.76	3.70	5.19	4.03			
*Perceptual Examination (total errors)	SF	7.92	7.74	8.42	9.18	.011 F = 6.76	.024 F = 3.85	n.s. F = 1.96
	SI	13.40	12.13	18.43	19.34			
	NSI	12.33	18.52	14.83	20.02			
*Name writing (letters/second written)	SF	.83	.27	1.04	.32	.001 F = 19.28	.001 F = 9.09	.001 F = 12.77
	SI	.70	.30	.87	.37			
	NSI	.70	.22	.63	.24			
*Category Test (errors)	SF	38.77	25.71	27.56	19.44	.001 F = 21.11	.026 F = 3.77	n.s. F = 2.26
	SI	50.13	31.76	39.80	27.98			
	NSI	49.12	26.04	46.56	31.66			
*Tactual Performance Test (total time)	SF	20.13	12.61	14.88	9.34	.001 F = 11.53	n.s. F = 2.83	n.s. F = 2.88
	SI	25.54	15.15	20.84	13.79			
	NSI	22.03	11.74	22.21	12.06			
*Tactual Performance Test, Memory (number of blocks remembered)	SF	7.19	1.43	7.47	1.30	n.s. F = 1.21	n.s. F = 1.62	n.s. F = 2.84
	SI	6.87	1.98	6.63	1.98			
	NSI	7.30	1.49	6.74	1.79			
*Tactual Performance Test, localisation (number of blocks localised)	SF	3.43	2.40	3.53	2.38	n.s. F = 1.65	n.s. F = 1.04	n.s. F = 0.95
	SI	3.53	2.19	3.03	2.12			
	NSI	2.96	2.44	2.52	2.23			
*Seashore Rhythm Test (items correct)	SF	24.62	3.80	25.08	3.34	n.s. F = 0.37	.005 F = 5.48	n.s. F = 2.38
	SI	22.03	4.48	23.27	3.96			
	NSI	23.08	3.77	22.36	3.53			

Table 4 continued on next page

Table 4. *(continued)* A comparison of pre-operative vs. post-operative performances on the WAIS and on selected variables of the Neuropsychological Battery for Epilepsy across seizure relief groups.

Test variable		Before surgery		At 5/10 yr. follow-up		Statistical significance		
		M	SD	M	SD	Over time	Across seizure relief groups	Time x group interaction
*Seashore Tonal Memory Test (items correct)	SF	20.74	6.88	21.09	6.62	n.s. F = 0.37	n.s. F = 2.84	n.s. F = 0.86
	SI	19.23	6.98	19.10	7.15			
	NSI	17.68	6.87	16.64	7.45			
*Finger Tapping, total (taps/10 seconds)	SF	92.00	12.91	98.21	13.10	.001 F = 27.96	.003 F = 5.85	n.s. F = 1.48
	SI	88.34	17.42	91.24	17.96			
	NSI	84.58	16.09	88.19	16.18			
Trail Making Test, Part A (seconds)	SF	30.87	15.46	25.42	15.60	n.s. F = 0.02	.008 F = 5.00	.005 F = 5.56
	SI	40.93	19.14	36.07	22.00			
	NSI	41.24	27.70	50.68	55.74			
*Trail Making Test, Part B (seconds)	SF	84.70	54.94	67.85	39.47	n.s. F = 0.03	.002 F = 6.53	.002 F = 6.64
	SI	103.90	68.48	99.00	69.07			
	NSI	115.84	67.09	135.32	82.36			
*Aphasia Screening Test (total errors)	SF	2.72	2.57	2.38	3.22	n.s. F = 0.24	n.s. F = 2.50	.004 F = 5.73
	SI	4.30	3.54	3.03	2.92			
	NSI	3.92	6.28	5.12	6.39			
*Constructional Dyspraxia (degree of distortion in drawings)	SF	1.08	.85	.91	.82	n.s. F = 0.41	.028 F = 3.69	n.s. F = 0.51
	SI	1.37	1.03	1.37	.93			
	NSI	1.44	1.00	1.44	.87			
Summary measure: % of 16 tests outside normal limits	SF	47.85	28.59	35.87	25.25	n.s. F = 3.54	.001 F = 8.07	.001 F = 11.38
	SI	59.17	28.57	58.17	29.34			
	NSI	62.04	19.34	66.36	25.32			

NOTE: SF = Seizure-free (with or without auras) in the final two years of follow-up (n = 57); SI = Significantly Improved (at least a 75% reduction in seizures during the final two years of follow-up in comparison with the preoperative seizure rate for the two years prior to surgery; n = 30); NSI = Not Significantly Improved (less than a 75% reduction in seizure rate since surgery; n = 25). WAIS = Wechsler Adult Intelligence Scale. WMS (1) = Wechsler Memory Scale (Form 1). (*) indicates one of the 16 test variables in the Neuropsychological Battery for Epilepsy (Dodrill, 1978) the results of which are compiled together as the Summary measure.

even if this is not always seen in the available probability levels. Going down the 'Over time' column, for example, shows that the WAIS Performance IQ has far greater practice effects than any other variable. Perusing the 'Across seizure relief groups' column shows that the most reliable underlying difference across the seizure relief groups is to be found on the Stroop Test (speed of reading of words), the Name Writing procedure (speed of writing), and the Summary measure (percent of 16 tests outside normal limits). For the 'Time by group interaction' effect, these same neuropsychological tests are again among those showing the closest relationships, but on this occasion, the WAIS Verbal IQ score (and, consequently Full Scale IQ) show an even closer relationship. In fact, on the majority of test measures, cognitive changes were tied to seizure relief. Also, considering all the test variables together, it appears that indeed changes in verbal cognitive abilities are slightly more related to changes in seizure relief than are changes in visual-spatial functions. Improvements in seizure frequency are related in degree to improvements on these selected tests. Likewise, when there was not an improvement in seizure frequency which exceeded 75% on a long-term basis, performances on the cognitive tests were either the same or slightly worse.

The results of the study just reported seem to go farther and to be more definitive than the results of most of the studies detailed in Table 3. Having three seizure relief outcome groups appeared to be helpful here as well as having a broad battery of neuropsychological tests that went beyond areas such as intelligence and memory to reveal additional relationships that would otherwise not have been found. However, the results of the present study did not usually contradict those of previous studies, but rather they extended the previously reported findings. Verbally mediated tasks, especially when timed, seem to be more tightly linked to relief from seizures following surgery for epilepsy, whereas visual-spatial abilities, motor functions, and basic overall intactness of brain functions (Category Test, Tactual Performance Test, Seashore Rhythm and Tonal Memory Tests) are not consistently related to relief from seizures.

Studies of non-surgical patients

The focus here has been on surgical patients simply because they are the most likely to show a great change in seizure frequency so that the cognitive correlates of that change might be evaluated. However, with the removal of parts of the brain, there can obviously be complicating factors, especially if viable tissue has been removed and the seizure focus has been largely missed so that the seizures continue. Therefore, a model resulting in significant changes in seizure frequency but without the complicating factors of surgery would be desirable.

Treatment with antiepileptic drugs is the second obvious model to be considered, but it has its own drawbacks including the cognitive effects of the medications themselves. In addition, however, and of great importance is the fact that most medications do not result in dramatic reductions in seizure frequency in groups of patients. A seizure rate improvement of 25-50% is about the best that can be found in drug study groups, but as can be seen from the original investigation reported above, clear cognitive improvements may not be expected until seizure improvement exceeds 75%. Thus, studies of most or all drugs do not appear to be a source of good information about cognitive changes *when one wishes to study seizure relief in and of itself* rather than the intrinsic cognitive correlates of the drugs in question. Likewise other methods of inducing changes in seizure frequency (vagus nerve stimulator, behavioural modification, etc.) do not have a record of resulting in sufficient relief from seizures that cognitive change can be adequately assessed. Thus, no effort will be made here to evaluate studies arising from such approaches.

CONCLUSIONS

This chapter has shown that persisting seizures, especially tonic-clonic seizures, are associated with a decrease in mental abilities over time. These decreases are more evident in children than in adults, and they are most likely to be seen when the temporal pattern of attacks is one of closely occurring attacks (status epilepticus). Similar losses with partial seizures are more difficult to document although it is possible that some such losses do occur.

This chapter has also shown that relief from seizures is associated with favourable cognitive change that is related to the degree of seizure relief experienced, with more seizure relief associated with greater cognitive improvement. However, using a surgical model, such change does not appear reliably until there has been at least a 75% relief from seizures. Also, the change is not seen in an even way across mental abilities. Verbally mediated tasks, especially when timed, seem to be more tightly linked to relief from seizures following surgery for epilepsy, whereas visual-spatial abilities, motor functions, and basic overall intactness of brain functions are not as consistently related to relief from seizures.

Taken as a whole, the presence of seizures, and their subsequent absence, does have an impact upon cognitive functions. While that impact is complex by nature, the overall finding here is another encouragement to us to do everything that we can to rid our patients of seizures. Let us all redouble our efforts towards this end.

REFERENCES

Aikia, M. and Kalviainen, R. (1999). Five-year follow-up of cognitive performance of adult patients with well-controlled partial epilepsy. *Epilepsia* **40(suppl 2)**, 100-101.

Aldenkamp, A.P., Alpherts, W.C.J., Bruine-Seeder, D.D. and Dekker, M.J.A. (1990). Test-retest variability in children with epilepsy—a comparison of WISC-R profiles. *Epilepsy Research* **7**, 165-172.

Arieff, A.J., Yacorzynski G.K. (1942). Deterioration of patients with organic epilepsy. *J Nerv Ment Dis* **96**, 49-55.

Binder L.M., Storzbach, D., Anger, W.K., Campbell, K.A., Rohlman, D.S., and other members of the Portland Environmental Hazards Research Center. (1999). Subjective cognitive complaints, affective distress, and objective cognitive performance in Persian Gulf War Veterans. *Arch Clin Neuropsychol* **14**, 531-536.

Bjornaes, H., Stabell, K., Henriksen, O. and Loyning, Y. (2001). The effects of refractory epilepsy on intellectual functioning in children and adults. A longitudinal study. *Seizure* **210**, 250-259.

Bourgeois, B.F.D., Prensky, A.L., Palkes, H.S., Talent, B.K. and Buxch, S.G. (1983). Intelligence in epilepsy: a prospective study in children. Ann Neurol **14**, 438-444.

Cañizares, S., Torres, X., Boget, T., Rumià, J., Elices, E., and Arroyo, S. (2000). Does neuroticism influence cognitive self-assessment after epilepsy surgery? *Epilepsia* **41**, 1303-1309.

Dawson, S. and Conn, J.C.M. (1929). The intelligence of epileptic children. *Arch Dis Childhood* **4**, 142-151.

Dodrill, C. B. (1978). A Neuropsychological Battery for Epilepsy. *Epilepsia* **19**, 611-623.

Dodrill, C.B. Progressive cognitive decline in adolescents and adults with epilepsy. (2000). In: Sutula, T. and Pitkänen, A. (Eds), Do seizures damage the brain? *Prog in Brain Res* **135**, 399-407.

Dodrill, C.B. (2002). Progressive decline in adolescents and adults with epilepsy. In: Sutula, T. and Pitkänen, A. (Eds), Do seizures damage the brain? *Prog in Brain Res* **135**, 399-407.

Dodrill, C.B. and Wilensky, A.J. (1992). Neuropsychological abilities before and after 5 years of stable antiepileptic drug therapy. *Epilepsia* **33**, 327-334.

Dodrill, C.B. and Wilensky, A.J. (1990). Intellectual impairment as an outcome of status epilepticus. *Neurology* **40(suppl 2)**, 23-27.

Ellenberg, J.H., Hirtz, D.G. and Nelson, K.B. (1986). Do seizures in children cause intellectual deterioration? *N Engl J Med* **314**, 1085-1088.

Fetterman, J. and Barnes, M.R. (1934). Serial studies of the intelligence of patients with epilepsy. *Arch Neurol Psychiat* **32**, 797-801.

Fox, J.T. (1924). The response of epileptic children to mental and educational tests. *Brit J Med Psychol* **4**, 235-248.

Gass, C.S. and Apple, C. (1997). Cognitive complaints in closed-head injury: Relationship to memory test performance and emotional disturbance. *J Clin Exper Neuropsychol* **19**, 290-299.

Helmstaedter, C., Kurthen, M., Lux, S., Reuber, M., Elger, C.E. (2003). Chronic epilepsy and cognition: a longitudinal study in temporal lobe epilepsy. *Ann Neurol* **54,** 425-432.

Helmstaedter, C., Kurthen, M.., Lux, S., Johanson, K., Quiske, A., Schramm, J. and Elger, C.E. (2000). Temporal lobe epilepsy: longitudinal clinical, neuropsychological and psychosocial follow-up of surgically and conservatively managed patients. *Nervenarzt*; **71**, 629-642. (German).

Holmes, M.D., Dodrill, C.B., Wilkus, R.J., Ojemann, L.M. and Ojemann, G.A. (1998). Is partial epilepsy progressive? Ten-year follow-up of EEG and neuropsychological changes in adults with partial seizures. *Epilepsia* **39**, 1189-1193.

Kalska, H. (1991) Cognitive changes in epilepsy: a ten-year follow-up. *Commentationes Scientiarum Socialium* **44**, 1-85. Societas Scientiarum Fennica, Helsinki.

Lieb, J.P., Rausch, R., Engel, Jr. J, Brown W.J., and Crandall, P.H. (1982). Changes in intelligence following temporal lobectomy: relationship to EEG activity, seizure relief, and pathology. *Epilepsia* **23**, 1-13.

Lineweaver, T.T., Naugle, R.I., Cafaro, A.M., Bingaman, W. and Lüders, H.O. (2004). Patients' perceptions of memory functioning before and after surgical intervention to treat medically refractory epilepsy. *Epilepsia* **45**, 1604-1612.

Matarazzo, J.D. (1972). *Wechsler's Measurement and Appraisal of Adult Intelligence 5th edn.* Williams and Wilkins, Baltimore.

McGlone, J. (1994). Memory complaints before and after temporal lobectomy: Do they predict memory performance or lesion laterality. *Epilepsia* **35**, 529-539.

Novelly, R.A., Augustine, E.A., Mattson, R.H., Glaser, G.H, Williamson, P.D., Spencer, D. D., and Spencer, S.S. (1984). Selective memory improvement and impairment in temporal lobectomy for epilepsy. *Ann Neurol* **15**, 64-67.

Patterson, H.A. and Fonner, D. (1928). Some observations on the intelligence quotient in epileptics. *Psychiat Quar* **2**, 542-548.

Reitan, R.M. and Wolfson, D. (1993). *The Halstead-Reitan Neuropsychological Test Battery*. Tucson: Neuropsychology Press.

Rodin, E.A. (1968). *The Prognosis of Patients with Epilepsy*. Charles C. Thomas, Springfield, Illinois.

Seidenberg, M., O'Leary, D.S., Berent, S. and Boll, T. (1981). Changes in seizure frequency and test-retest scores on the Wechsler Adult Intelligence Scale. *Epilepsia* **22**, 75-83.

Selwa, L.M., Berent, S., Giordan,i B., Henry, T.R., Buchtel, H.A. and Ross, D.A. (1994). Serial cognitive testing in temporal lobe epilepsy: longitudinal changes with medical and surgical therapies. *Epilepsia* **35**, 743-749.

Sullivan, E.B. and Gahagan, L. (1935). On intelligence of epileptic children. *Genetic Psychology Monographs* **17**, 309-375.

Sutula, T. and Pitkanen, A. (2002). (Eds), Do seizures damage the brain? *Prog in Brain Res* **135**, 1-520.

Vercoulen, J.H.M.M., Bazelmans, E., Swanink C.M.A., Galama, J.M.D., Fennis, J.F.M, van der Meer, J.W.M.. and Bleijenberg G. (1998). Evaluating neuropsychological impairment in chronic fatigue syndrome. *J Clin Exper Neuropsychol* **20**, 144-156.

Vingerhoets, G. (1998). Cognitive, emotional and psychosomatic complaints and their relation to emotional status and personality following cardiac surgery. *Brit J Health Psychol* **3**, 159-169.

Seizure Freedom: Clinical, Research and Quality of Life Perspectives
Edited by Michael R. Trimble
© 2006 Clarius Press Ltd

11

Epilepsy and Driving

MASSIMILIANO BEGHI[1] and ETTORE BEGHI[2]

[1]*Department of Psychiatry,*
University of Milano-Bicocca, Ospedale 'San Gerardo',
Monza, Italy

[2]*Department of Neurology,*
Istituto di Ricerche Farmacologiche 'Mario Negri',
Milano, Italy

INTRODUCTION

Epilepsy is a clinical condition characterised by repeated unprovoked seizures (Commission, 1993). In the adult population, the prevalence of active epilepsy, namely, persistent seizures and / or continuing anticonvulsant treatment, is about 4-10/1000 (Hauser *et al.*, 1996). For their adverse effects on daily living activities, recurring seizures lead to the lack of driving privileges, which is one of the major concerns of people with epilepsy. A recent epidemiological study conducted in seven western and eastern European countries (RESt-1 Group, 2000) confirms that fewer adult patients with epilepsy hold a driving licence compared to the general population (31% vs 43%). This is an important limitation in the patient's life activities because, without a driving licence, it is difficult to be mobile, to be employed, and to be a full participant in all aspects of daily living. However, the heterogeneity of epilepsy and the differing liability to seizure remission and relapse are a pre-requisite for considering driving restrictions from a more complex perspective. In order to give a better understanding of the real influence of the disease on driving restrictions, the overall issue of epilepsy and driving must be subjected to a critical view and the following issues must be addressed:

    a. methodological issues in studies on epilepsy and driving;

    b. European legislation for driving and epilepsy;

    c. fraction of accidents and injuries attributable to epilepsy and seizures;

    d. clinical heterogeneity of epilepsy and seizures, and differing liability to seizure relapse;

    e. risk of seizure-related accidents and injuries in people with epilepsy by disease type and severity; and

    f. factors influencing the ability to drive in people with epilepsy.

These different points will be discussed in the following sections.

METHODOLOGICAL ISSUES IN STUDIES ON EPILEPSY AND DRIVING

A correct assessment of the accident rate in drivers with epilepsy is virtually impossible. The estimation of seizure frequency in people with epilepsy is, with few exceptions, based on the patients' reports and not by laboratory tests or the physician's own observations. A study from the United Kingdom (Dalrymple and Appleby, 2000) compared seizure frequency as referred by the patients to their general practitioner with that reported in a linked anonymous questionnaire. According to the questionnaire, 40% of interviewees had had a seizure in the past year, but only 10% of them reported the seizure to their doctor.

In the United Kingdom all drivers are required to inform the driving licence agency about any symptom or diagnosis that may relate to their medical fitness to drive. However, Taylor and colleagues (1995) found that less than one third of the patients with newly diagnosed epilepsy or other unexplained episodes of loss of consciousness returned the compulsory notification slip to the authorities. In other countries, such as Sweden, the responsibility to inform the authorities that the driver is no longer fit to drive lies primarily with the treating physician (Tomson *et al.*, 2004). There are no studies reporting on how physicians fulfil this obligation. The under-reporting of epilepsy or seizure frequency from patients and physicians is a possible source of selection bias in studies on accident rates in people with epilepsy.

EUROPEAN LEGISLATION FOR DRIVING AND EPILEPSY

Current laws in most countries permit epilepsy patients with controlled seizures to drive. These laws attempt to balance the important economic and social value of driving with the risk to public safety from seizure-related crashes. Various clinical factors are considered, but the length of the prescribed seizure-free interval is the dominating factor. The European Council Directive 91/439/EEC on driving licences reports that *'a licence may be issued or renewed subject to an examination by a competent medical authority and to regular medical check ups. The authority shall decide on the state of the epilepsy or other disturbances of consciousness, its clinical form and*

Table 1. Driving regulations for people with epilepsy in the European Union by country and category

Country	Group	N of months seizure-free	Exceptions/Notes
United Kingdom	I	12	Seizures during sleep, with pattern established by year 3.
	II	120	They must have not taken drugs for this 10-year period, after a medical examination. Risk should be less than 2% per annum.
France	I	12	Seizures only on awakening or during sleep. First unprovoked seizure: 6 months.
	II	60	First unprovoked seizure; 36 months.
Germany	I	12	Single seizure or occasion-related seizures: 3-6 months; first idiopathic seizure: 3-6 months; discontinuation of treatment: 3 months .
	II	60 (no drugs)	First idiopathic seizure: 24 months.
Netherlands	I	12	First unprovoked seizure and sporadic seizures: 6 months; first idiopathic seizure, myoclonias, simple partial seizures, discontinuation of treatment: 3 months.
	II	60 (no drugs and 3 normal EEGs)	First unprovoked seizure, untreated and no epileptiform EEG abnormalities: 2 years.
Belgium	I	12	First unprovoked seizure: 6 months; seizures not interfering with driving: 3 months; seizures exclusively in sleep: pattern should be established for 24 months.
	II	120 (no drugs and normal EEG)	First unprovoked seizure: 5 years; first provoked seizure: 2 years.
Italy	I	24	Validity for two years.
	II	Prohibited	None.
Spain	I	12	First unprovoked seizure: 6 months; seizures exclusively in sleep: pattern should be established for 12 months.
	II	60 (no drugs)	First unprovoked seizure: 12 months.
Ireland	I	12	Seizures during sleep: pattern should be established for 12 months.
	II	prohibited	None.
Portugal	I	24	Nocturnal seizures, simple partial seizures, favourable neurological report.
	II	Prohibited	None.

Table 1 continued on next page

Table 1. *(continued)* Driving regulations for people with epilepsy in the European Union by country and category

Country	Group	N of months seizure-free	Exceptions/Notes
Slovenia	I	24	Seizures during sleep.
	II	Prohibited	Distant seizure history.
Croatia	I	24	People who are taking drugs contraindicated with driving are not allowed to drive.
Finland	I	12	First unprovoked seizure with normal tests: 3 months; sporadic seizures (3-year interval): 6 months; myoclonias: able to drive.
	II	Prohibited	None.
Greece	I	24	None.
Sweden	I	24	Single unprovoked seizure: 12 months Seizures in sleep; seizures without influence on driving; sporadic seizures; seizures after change of medication.
	II	60 (with taxis)	Seizures in sleep; seizures without influence on driving; sporadic seizures; seizures after change of medication and nocturnal seizures.
Norway	I	12	Seizures after change in medication and nocturnal seizures.
	II	120 (with taxis)	Seizures after change in medication and nocturnal seizures.
Switzerland	I	12	Complex partial seizures; sleep seizures established for 3 years, avoidable reflex seizures; treatment discontinuation: 3 months; first unprovoked seizure: 6 months; first provoked seizure: 2 months; single relapse after 2-year seizure freedom: 3 months.
	II	60 (no drugs)	None.
Denmark	I	24	Seizures during sleep, licence valid for 1 year, 2 years if patient is seizure-free for >2 years, 5 years if patient is seizure-free for >4 years.
	II	120 (buses 240)	Off drugs for 5 years.
Estonia	I	24	None.
	II	prohibited	None.
Lithuania	I +II	prohibited	None.
Austria	I	12	Epilepsy of long duration and difficult to treat: 18 months.
	II	prohibited	None.

I = Non-commercial; II = Commercial;

progress (no seizure in the last two years, for example), the treatment received and the results thereof' (Council Directive, 1991). For commercial driving it states *'driving licences shall not be issued for applicants or drivers suffering or liable to suffer from epileptic seizures or other sudden disturbances of the state of consciousness.'*

Drivers can be divided in two different groups. Group I refers to motor-bikes and cars, Group II refers to lorries and buses. Taxi drivers may be included in Group I or II, the decision being taken country by country. For Group I, a licence could be issued or renewed subject to an examination by a competent medical authority and to regular medical check-ups. The authority would decide on the state of epilepsy or other disturbances of consciousness, their clinical form and progress, the treatments received and the results thereof. For Group II, driving licences would not be issued to or renewed for applicants or drivers suffering or liable to suffer from epileptic seizures or other sudden disturbances of the state of consciousness. In the European Union, some member states, including the United Kingdom, require a one-year period of freedom from seizures before granting or renewing a driving licence although most require a two-year period (Table 1). All these issues have been dealt with in a review paper (Schmedding, 2004) and have been discussed in a recent comprehensive scientific report on epilepsy and driving in Europe, prepared by the advisory board to the driving licence committee of the European Union (Second European Working Group on Epilepsy and Driving, 2005).

Compared to the European rules, in the United States the regulations are less severe and differ significantly among the individual states (Fisher *et al.*, 1994).

FRACTION OF ACCIDENTS AND INJURIES ATTRIBUTABLE TO EPILEPSY AND SEIZURES

On average, a European citizen with a driving licence spends 4% of his/her lifetime behind the wheel (60 min per day) (European Commission Transport Internet Site). By contrast, a professional driver typically spends up to eight hours per working day behind the wheel, which is about 20% of his/her lifetime, which is six times as long as car drivers.

Data from the Netherlands (Second European Working Group on Epilepsy and Driving, 2005) suggest that driving a car is one of the least dangerous forms of road use compared to driving a moped (which in some countries does not require driving licence) or being a cyclist, which are 3-25 times more dangerous per kilometer driven. Sonnen (1997) calculated the risk of accidents from a seizure for different vehicles. He attributed factors of severity to four items, which include driving time, toll of accidents, seizure accident ratio, and passenger transport. For taxis, ambulances and lorries, the risk seems considerably lower than for buses. Minibuses have an intermediate risk. The risk for taxi drivers is not really known. Taxi drivers often spend several hours behind the wheel, but much of it is waiting for costumers. On the other hand, in some countries or cities, taxi drivers drive around all the time. Here, the number of kilometers behind the wheel increases and also the risk for seizure-related traffic accidents increases. Motorbikes should be assessed more critically than cars, as an accident represents a two to three times greater danger for the driver (Second European Working Group on Epilepsy and Driving, 2005).

In this context, the proportion of accidents attributable to active epileptic seizures is extremely low, ranging from 0.02% to 0.2% (Black *et al.*, 1997; Sheth *et al.*, 2004) and compares favourably with other causes. In a population-based US study of traffic deaths, alcohol abuse (31%), young age (24%) and cardiac and hypertensive disorders (4%) were among the leading causes of death (Sheth *et al.*, 2004). In this study, epilepsy-related accidents (0.2%) constituted a small minority of all fatal car crashes. According to Parsonage (1992), epilepsy-related accidents are 1/400. Only 1/250 hospital admissions after a traffic accident have been shown to have an associated medical factor (Taylor *et al.*, 1996). Of these, 37% were associated with seizures. Fifteen percent of these accidents were caused by first seizures and were thus unavoidable.

In a recent study done in the state of Arizona, US (Drazkowski, 2003), the number of motor vehicle crashes related to seizures, other medical conditions, and other non-medical crashes was calculated comparing the three years before and the three years after the legal reduction of the seizure-free driving interval from 12 months to three months. Seizure-related crashes did not increase after the reduction of the seizure-free interval.

In summary, traffic accidents attributable to epileptic seizures represent a small fraction of the overall number of traffic accidents and are far behind other putative causes, like young age, recreational drugs (alcohol), or other clinical conditions (cardiovascular disorders).

CLINICAL HETEROGENEITY OF EPILEPSY AND SEIZURES, AND DIFFERING LIABILITY TO SEIZURE RELAPSE

While all people with epilepsy experience seizures, not all individuals with seizures have epilepsy. Epileptic seizures may be unprovoked or they may occur in the context of a brain insult (systemic, toxic or metabolic) (Commission, 1993). Unprovoked seizures include idiopathic or cryptogenic seizures, caused by an as yet undetected disease or factor, and remote symptomatic seizures, occurring in patients with a static encephalopathy. In contrast, provoked or acute symptomatic seizures are presumed to be an acute manifestation of a CNS insult and may not recur when the underlying cause has been removed or the acute phase has elapsed. In a meta-analysis of 16 prospective studies (Berg and Shinnar, 1991) the authors found a relapse rate of 40% at one year after a first seizure. The pooled recurrence risk in patients with a first idiopathic/cryptogenic seizure was 32% (95% CI 28-35%) as compared to 57% (95% CI 51-63%) with a remote symptomatic seizure. The recurrence risk ranged from 27% (95% CI 21-33%) with a normal EEG tracing to 58% (95% CI 49-66%) with an EEG showing epileptiform abnormalities. Seizures occurring during sleep tend to be associated with a higher risk of recurrence both in children and in adults (Hopkins et al., 1988; van Donselaar et al., 1991). Partial seizures, which are mostly associated with a documented brain injury, are also correlated with a higher risk of recurrent seizures, even after controlling for aetiology and EEG abnormalities (Annegers et al., 1986). On the other hand, after a second seizure, this risk is about 70% (Hauser et al., 1998). The risk is 32% after three months, 53% after six months, 68% after one year, and 87% after two years.

Although epilepsy is, by definition, a chronic clinical condition, about two-thirds of patients achieve seizure remission, most immediately after treatment initiation (Forsgren, 2004). Moreover, population-based studies on the long-term prognosis of treated epilepsy report a 58-65% cumulative 5-year remission rate at 10 years (Annegers et al., 1979; Cockerell et al., 1997).

The aetiology of epilepsy is by far the strongest prognostic predictor for seizure recurrence. In general, idiopathic epilepsy has a better chance of seizure remission than symptomatic or cryptogenic epilepsy. In the population of Rochester, Minnesota, symptomatic epilepsies have been found to achieve a significantly lower chance of 5-year remission compared to idiopathic epilepsies (30 vs. 42% at 15 years) (Annegers et al., 1979). Within this group, patients with neurological dysfunction present at birth had the lowest chance of remission (46% and 30% off-drugs at 20 years). Lower, albeit less significant, remission rates in patients with symptomatic epilepsies were also found in the United Kingdom, Sweden (adults) and Finland (adults with childhood-onset epilepsy) (Jallon, 2003).

Other indicators of 5-year remission in the Rochester, Minnesota population, included absence of EEG epileptiform abnormalities and absence of generalized tonic-clonic seizures (Shafer et al., 1988). In the National General Practice Study of Epilepsy (NGPSE), the only independent predictor of 1-year and 2-year remission was the number of seizures experienced by the patient after the first seizure (Cockerell et al., 1997; MacDonald et al., 2000). When other prognostic predictors are excluded, there is no evidence that age at onset of seizures affects seizure outcome. With the exception of rare inherited sex-linked disorders, sex has not been indicated as a significant prognostic predictor.

In a long-term retrospective population-based study, 5-year terminal remission (i.e. off drugs) of epilepsy was 61% (Annegers *et al.*, 1979). Discontinuation of drug treatment is thus a valuable option in patients with epilepsy who are seizure-free for two years or longer. In a critical review of 28 studies including 4,615 patients with epilepsy (2,802 children and 1,020 adults), most of whom had at least two years of seizure remission, the proportion of individuals with relapses during or after treatment withdrawal ranged from 12 to 66% (Specchio and Beghi, 2004). The cumulative probability of remaining seizure-free in adults was 39-74% at one year, and 35-57% at two years. The relapse rate was highest in the first 12 months (especially in the first six months) and tended to decrease thereafter. In a meta-analysis of 25 studies, the pooled relapse risk was 25% (95% CI, 21-30%) at one year and 29% (95% CI, 24-34%) at two years (Berg and Shinnar, 1994).

A number of factors have been associated with favourable or unfavourable seizure outcome after treatment discontinuation. As shown by a recent systematic review (Specchio and Beghi, 2004), factors consistently indicating a higher risk of seizure relapse include adolescent-onset epilepsy, partial seizures, presence of an underlying neurological condition, and abnormal EEG findings (children). Factors associated with a lower risk were childhood epilepsy, idiopathic generalised epilepsy, and – for children – a normal EEG. Selected epilepsy syndromes (e.g. benign epilepsy with centro-temporal spikes and juvenile myoclonic epilepsy) may be associated with significantly different outcomes after treatment withdrawal.

In summary, the overall prognosis of epilepsy is favourable in the majority of cases, with about 50 to 70% of newly diagnosed patients achieving seizure remission. The average recurrence risk of a first unprovoked seizure is about 50%, with half of recurrences occurring during the first six months. Risk factors for recurrence include a documented aetiology, an abnormal EEG, a partial seizure, and a seizure occurring during sleep. Factors influencing the prognosis of epilepsy include aetiology, EEG abnormalities, generalized tonic-clonic seizures, the number of seizures experienced at the onset of treatment, and the syndromic pattern. The average risk of relapse after treatment discontinuation in seizure-free patients is 25% at one year and about 30% at two years. Predictors of seizure relapse include aetiology, EEG abnormalities at time of ending treatment, and epilepsy syndrome.

RISK OF SEIZURE-RELATED ACCIDENTS AND INURIES IN PEOPLE WITH EPILEPSY BY DISEASE TYPE AND SEVERITY

The role of seizures as a potential risk factor for accidents and injuries has been assessed in several epidemiological investigations. In a population-based retrospective cohort study of 30,420 subjects including all the licensed drivers from seven contiguous ZIP Code areas in Wisconsin, US, with and without epilepsy or diabetes mellitus, the traffic accident ratio was 1.33 (p=0.04) for epilepsy and 1.32 (p=0.01) for diabetes (Hansotia and Broste, 1991). In a retrospective study from the United Kingdom comparing self-completed questionnaires from 16,958 drivers (who had notified the authorities about a single epileptic seizure or diagnosed epilepsy) and 8,888 normal drivers, no overall differences were found in total accident rate, but serious injuries were increased by 40% in people with epilepsy, with a 2-fold increase in non-driver fatalities (Taylor et al., 1996). In a Danish study (Lings, 2001) done in a 10-year historical cohort register including 159 patients with epilepsy and 559 controls matched for age, gender, place of residence, and exposure period, the accident rate per 1,000 person-years was 7.0 (95% CI 2.2-26.1) in patients with epilepsy.

Several factors are associated with increased or decreased odds of traffic accidents in patients with epilepsy. Gastaut and Zifkin (1987) reported 97 patients having 109 seizures while driving. Fifty-five percent of these seizures led to a traffic accident. The risk varied with seizure type (complex partial seizures without aura and tonic-clonic seizures 75%; complex partial seizures with aura 33%). A retrospective case-control study of accident rates in outpatients attending an epilepsy clinic (Krauss et al., 1999) identified clinical risk factors for seizure-related motor vehicle crashes in patients with epilepsy. Both case and control patients had epilepsy, drove, and were from the same clinic, but the index cases differed from the controls in the number of seizure-related motor vehicle crashes. Factors significantly decreasing the odds of seizure-related crashes in people with epilepsy included long seizure-free intervals, reliable auras, fewer prior non seizure-related accidents, and a reduction or switch of anti-epileptic drugs. Patients who had a seizure-free interval $\geq$12 months had a 93% reduced odds for crashing compared to patients with shorter intervals. Twenty-five percent of patients had more than one seizure-related crash and 20% had missed an AED dose just prior to their crash. The majority (54%) of patients who crashed were driving illegally, with seizure-free intervals shorter than legally permitted.

Berg and colleagues (2000) interviewed a group of 367 patients included in an epilepsy surgery programme and found that one third of them drove regularly, despite having frequent seizures. In this study, 115 (31.3%) had driven in the last year, most on at least a weekly basis. Factors associated with an increased likelihood of driving were having a current licence (OR = 10.7, p < 0.001), ever having had a licence (OR = 3.9, p = 0.003), and being younger. By contrast, people who were less likely to drive included women (OR = 0.3, p < 0.001), individuals self-described as disabled (OR = 0.2, p < 0.001), and people who were employed full-time (OR = 0.4, p = 0.03) or part-time (OR = 0.15, p = 0.005). Thirty-nine percent of patients had experienced one or more seizures while driving, and 27% at least one seizure-related accident. Of those who had accidents, 94% reported property damage, 32% had a self-injury, and 20% caused injury to others.

In a multicentre prospective European cohort study (Van den Broek and Beghi, 2004), the risk for street accidents, almost all of them traffic accidents, at 12 and 24 months was significantly higher for patients (5% and 7%) compared with controls (2% and 4%) (p<0.001). After exclusion of seizure-related events, the risk decreased to 4% at 12 months and 6% at 24 months, although it remained higher compared with controls (p<0.05). A possible explanation given by the authors is that part of this risk, although not easily quantifiable, may be attributed to the adverse effects of medications. Likewise, as indicated above, changes in treatment schedules have been reported in patients having road accidents (Krauss et al., 1999). With seizures, the effects of treatment can thus be considered a potential source of accidents in people with epilepsy.

In summary, the overall risk of seizure-related accidents in patients with active epilepsy might be high, with a pooled rate ratio of 1.8 (95% CI 1.7 to 2.0) (Vaa, 2003) and a moderately high risk of serious accidents (OR 1.4; 95% CI 1.0-1.8) (Taylor et al., 1996).

Fewer than half of all seizures, however, occur in the context of established epilepsy; the remainder consists of acute symptomatic seizures and single unprovoked seizures. Acute symptomatic seizures can be prevented by adequate control of the cause, whereas single unprovoked seizures have a smaller probability of relapse after the first 12 months (see above) (Hauser et al., 1998). Even among people with active epilepsy, several epilepsy syndromes exist (for example, nocturnal tonic-clonic epilepsy or epilepsies with simple partial seizures), which may be compatible with non-commercial driving.

FACTORS INFLUENCING THE ABILITY TO DRIVE IN PEOPLE WITH EPILEPSY

A number of factors have been identified by the Second European Working Group on Epilepsy and Driving as possibly affecting the ability to drive in people with epilepsy (Second European Working Group on Epilepsy and Driving, 2005). These factors are listed in Table 2. Some negative factors are disease- and patient-related and include, among others, young age, non-compliance, alcohol and/or drug abuse, the presence of a stable or non-correctable brain dysfunction, and seizure severity. In patients with seizures caused by chronic and/or non-correctable epileptogenic disorders, the degree of functional impairment caused by the underlying clinical condition should be properly evaluated.

Other negative factors are associated with the nature of the driving activity

Table 2. Factors associated to the ability to drive in people with epilepsy

Negative

A. Associated with patient's or disease characteristics

> Non-compliance with medication
> Alcohol/drug abuse in past 3 months
> Structural brain lesion
> Non-correctable brain functional/metabolic condition
> Periods of frequent seizures after seizure-free interval
> Severity of seizure

B. Associated with type of driving activity

> Driving a motorcycle
> Transport of passengers
> Driving considerable more hours than average
> Young age
> Nature of driving task (ie, transport of people, explosives, etc.)
> Other comorbid conditions (ie, diabetes, cardiovascular, etc.)
> Medications, especially multiple drugs

Positive

Provoked (acute symptomatic) seizures
Seizures during medically directed medication changes
Seizures not interfering with consciousness or motor control
Established pattern of pure nocturnal seizures

Source: Second European Working Group on Epilepsy and Driving, 2005

and comprise the use of more risky vehicles (like motorcycles), longer time at the wheel, and the nature of the driving task. Special attention should be directed to medication effects, which might be more intensive in people receiving multiple drug regimens and/or compounds with sedative effects.

By contrast, several factors have been found to decrease the chance of seizure-related accidents. These include preventable acute symptomatic seizures, seizures occurring during medication change or withdrawal, seizures not interfering with consciousness or with motor control, and pure nocturnal seizures.

A list of questions has been drawn up by Drachman (1999) to help physicians in assessing the driving capabilities in patients with epilepsy. These include:

a. the cause of the seizure experienced;
b. the means by which the condition is controlled (including medications and dosages);
c. the degree of impairment or disability suffered during a seizure;
d. the probability of seizure recurrence;

e. the date of the most recent seizure;

f. the certification, to a reasonable degree of medical certainty, that the individual's medical condition and medication will not interfere with the safe operation of a motor vehicle.

CONCLUSIONS

Despite the lack of population-based prospective data, there is strong evidence of an increase in traffic accidents in people with epilepsy. The preventive measures embedded in legislation, especially a prescribed seizure-free period before driving, are probably not observed by a substantial portion of people with epilepsy, and the extent to which physicians report their uncontrolled epilepsy patients to the authorities has not yet been elucidated. However, there are reasons to think that by making the law more liberal, more people will adhere to it (Sonnen, 1997; Krumholz *et al.*, 1991).

As recently suggested (Beghi and Sander, 2005), '... *an effort should be made by the driving authorities within the European Union to set common and more flexible rules considering epilepsy and seizures as a spectrum of clinical conditions, many of which are fully or partly compatible with non-commercial driving. Different periods of seizure freedom could be considered as a prerequisite for granting driving licences, depending on the type of epilepsy and seizure patterns. Acute symptomatic seizures should be considered separately, and may be compatible with non-commercial driving providing the underlying clinical condition is adequately identified and controlled. Likewise, patients with single unprovoked seizures should forego driving only for 12 months. In contrast, more strict rules should be set for commercial driving. Factors that determine risk of driving related accidents are the amount of time spent in driving, the number of previous accidents, and whether or not passengers are being transported (Sonnen, 1997). The driving authorities should consider these variables carefully when defining the length of the minimum seizure free period deemed necessary to grant or renew a driving licence.*'

If one accepts the concept that the risk is linked to time spent behind the wheel, restricting the time or distance driven will decrease the risk of accidents. One population-based study found that a restricted licensing programme appears to provide a significant decrease in the rate of crashes and traffic violations (Marshall *et al.*, 2002).

This can be an important alternative for people who are responsible enough and who cannot reach their work by other means of transport. Moreover, there are many factors linked with the ability to drive: these are often difficult to quantify. An individual assessment by a neurologist is recommended for every patient who has had one or more seizures.

ACKNOWLEDGEMENTS

The authors are indebted to Dr Eric Schmedding, Chair of the Second European Working Group on Epilepsy and Driving, for his precious help with the driving regulations in Europe.

REFERENCES

Annegers, J.F., Hauser, W.A. and Elveback, L.R. (1979). Remission of seizures and relapse in patients with epilepsy. *Epilepsia* **20**, 729-737.

Annegers, J.F., Shirts, S.B., Hauser, W.A. and Kurland, L.T. (1986). Risk of recurrence after an initial unprovoked seizure. *Epilepsia* **27**, 43-50.

Beghi, E. and Sander, J.W. (2005). Epilepsy and driving. *BMJ* **331**, 60-61.

Berg, A.T. and Shinnar, S. (1991). The risk of seizure recurrence following a first unprovoked seizure: a quantitative review. *Neurology* **41**, 965-972.

Berg, A.T. and Shinnar, S. (1994). Relapse following discontinuation of antiepileptic drugs: A meta-analysis. *Neurology* **44**, 601-608.

Berg, A.T., Vickrey, B.G., Sperling, M.R. et al. (2000). Driving in adults with refractory localisation-related epilepsy: multi-centre study of epilepsy surgery. *Neurology* **54**, 625-630.

Black, A.B. and Lai, N.Y. (1997). Epilepsy and driving in South Australia—an assessment of compulsory notification. *Med Law* **16**, 253-267.

Cockerell, O.C., Johnson, A.L. Sander, J.W.A.S. et al. (1997). Prognosis of Epilepsy: A Review and further analysis of the first nine years of the British National General Practice Study of Epilepsy, a prospective population-based study. *Epilepsia* **38**, 31-46.

Commission on Epidemiology and Prognosis. (1993). ILAE Guidelines for Epidemiologic Studies on Epilepsy. *Epilepsia* **34**, 592-596.

Council Directive 91/439/EEC of 29 July 1991 on driving licences. Official Journal L 237, 24/08/1991 P. 0001-0024. http://europa.eu.int/eur-lex/lex/LexUriServ/LexUriServ.do?uri=CELEX:31991L0439:EN:HTML.

Dalrymple, J. and Appleby, J. (2000). Cross sectional study of reporting of epileptic seizures to general practitioners. *BMJ* **320**, 94-97.

Drachman, D. (1999). Risk factors of seizure-related motor vehicle crashes in patients with epilepsy. *Neurology* **53**, 2214-2215.

Drazkowski, J.F., Fisher, R.S., Sirven, J.I. et al. (2003). Seizure-related motor vehicle crashes in Arizona before and after reducing the driving restrictions from 12 to 3 months. *Mayo Clin Proc* **78**, 819-825.

Fisher, R.S., Parsonage, M., Beaussart, M., et al. (1994). Epilepsy and driving: an international perspective. Joint Commission on Drivers' Licensing IBE / ILAE. *Epilepsia* **35**, 675-684.

Forsgren, L. (2004). Epidemiology and prognosis of epilepsy and its treatment. In: Fish, D., Dodson, E., Perucca, E and Shorvon, S. (Eds), *The Treatment of Epilepsy (2nd edition)*. Blackwell Science, Malden, MA, pp21-42.

Hauser, W.A., Annegers, J.F. and Rocca, W.A. (1996). Descriptive epidemiology of epilepsy: contributions of population-based studies from Rochester, Minnesota. *Mayo Clin Proc* **71**, 576-586.

Hauser, W.A., Rich, S.S., Lee, J.R-J. et al. (1998). Risk of recurrence after two unprovoked seizures. *N Eng J Med* **338**, 429-432.

Hansotia, P. and Broste, S.K. (1991). The effect of epilepsy or diabetes mellitus on the risk of automobile accidents. *N Engl J Med* **324**, 22-26.

Hopkins, A., Garman, A. and Clarke, C. (1988). The first seizure in adult life. Value of clinical features, electroencephalography, and computerised tomographic scanning in prediction of seizure recurrence. *Lancet* **1**, 721-726.

Jallon, P. (2003). *Prognosis of Epilepsies*. John Libbey Eurotext, Montrouge.

Krauss, G.I., Krumholz, A., Carter, R.C., Li, G. and Kaplan, P. (1999). Risk factors for seizure-related motor vehicle crashes in patients with epilepsy. *Neurology* **52**, 1324-1329.

Krumholz, A., Fisher, R.S., Lesser, R.P. and Hauser, W.A. (1991). Driving and epilepsy: a review and reappraisal. *JAMA* **265**, 622-626.

Lings, S. (2001). Increased driving accident frequency in Danish patients with epilepsy. *Neurology* **57**, 435-439.

MacDonald, B.K., Johnson, A.L., Goodridge, D.M. et al. (2000). Factors predicting prognosis of epilepsy after presentation with seizures. *Ann Neurol* **48**, 833-841.

Marshall, S.C., Spasoff, R., Nair, R., and van Walraven, C. (2002). Restricted driver licensing for medical impairments: does it work? *CMAJ* **167(7)**, 747-751.

Parsonage, M. (1992). *Epilepsy and driving licence regulations.* Report by the ILAE / IBE commission on drivers´ licensing; *IBE / ILAE* 1992. PO Box 21,210 AA Heemstede, The Netherlands.

RESt-1 Group (2000). Social aspects of epilepsy in the adult in seven European countries. *Epilepsia* **41**, 998-1004.

Schmedding, E. (2004). Epilepsy and driving in Belgium: proposals and justification. *Acta Neurol Belg* **104**, 68-79.

Second European Working Group on Epilepsy and Driving.(2005). *Epilepsy and Driving in Europe.* Http://europa.eu.int/comm./transport/home/drivinglicence/ fitnesstodrive/index_eu.htm, 2005.

Shafer, S.Q., Hauser, W.A., Annegers, J.F. and Klass, D.W. (1988). EEG and other early predictors of epilepsy remission: a community study. *Epilepsia* **29**, 590-600.

Sheth, S.G., Krauss, G., Krumholz, A. and Li, G. (2004). Mortality in epilepsy: driving fatalities vs other causes of death in patients with epilepsy. *Neurology* **63**, 1002-1007.

Sonnen A.E. and the European Working Group. (1995). *Epilepsy and Driving.* Proceedings First European Workshop epilepsy and Driving Licences Group 1. IBE May 1995.

Sonnen, A.E. (1997). *Epilepsy and driving: a European view.* International Bureau for Epilepsy. Paswerk Bedrijven, The Netherlands, pp11-32.

Specchio, L.M. and Beghi, E. (2004). Should antiepileptic drugs be withdrawn in seizure-free patients? *CNS Drugs* **18**, 201-212.

Taylor, J., Chadwick, D. and Johnson, T. (1995). Accident experiences and notification rates in people with recent seizures, epilepsy or undiagnosed episodes of loss of conciousness. *QJM* **88**, 733-740.

Taylor, J., Chadwick, D. and Johnson, T. (1996). Risk of accidents in drivers with epilepsy. *J Neurol Nurosurg Psychiatry* **60**, 621-627.

Tomson, T., Beghi, E., Sundqvist, A. and Johannessen, S.I. (2004). Medical risks in epilepsy: a review with focus on physical injuries, mortality, traffic accidents and their prevention. *Epilepsy Res* **60**, 1-16.

Vaa, T. (2003). Impairments, diseases, age and their relative risk of accident involvement: results from meta-analysis 2003. Report to the Institute of Transport Economics, PO Box 6110 Etterstad, N-0602 Oslo, Norway (www.toi.no/attach/a509491r891552/690_2003.pdf).

van den Broek, M. and Beghi, E. (2004). For the RESt-1 group. Accidents in patients with epilepsy: types, circumstances and complications: a European cohort study. *Epilepsia* **45**, 667-72.

van Donselaar, C.A., Geerts, A.T. and Schimsheimer, R.J. (1991). Idiopathic first seizure in adult life: who should be treated? *BMJ* **302**, 620-623.

12

Epilepsy and Quality of Life –
How Important is Seizure Freedom

GUS A. BAKER[1] and ANN JACOBY[2]

[1]*Clinical Science Centre for Research & Education,
Fazakerley, Liverpool, UK*

[2]*Division of Public Health, 3rd Floor, Wheelan Building,
Brownlow Hill, Liverpool, UK*

INTRODUCTION

In this chapter, we consider the relationship between seizure frequency and quality of life for people with epilepsy. We review available research evidence about the role of seizure frequency and other clinical variables in reducing quality of life; and about the way in which attaining complete freedom from seizures can promote quality of life. We will also consider reasons why the relationship between quality of life and seizure frequency is not necessarily a simple linear one and why even people with epilepsy who become seizure-free may continue to need support to maximise their life quality.

QUALITY OF LIFE AS A RELEVANT CONCEPT

The primary goal of medicine has always been to attempt to improve the quality of patients' lives, either by curing them of their disease or by ameliorating their symptoms. Consequently, doctors make implicit, if not explicit, quality of life (QOL) assessments when determining the most appropriate treatment for their patients. However, assessing the outcome of treatment has traditionally depended on clinical end points based on anatomical, physiological and biochemical markers, rather than on direct measures of quality of life; and it is only over the last two decades that there has been any general acknowledgment of the potential limits of such measures and their failure to address issues important to patients themselves as relevant to their day- to-day functioning. This important 'paradigm shift' has seen increasing emphasis on the need to describe outcomes of treatment in ways that make sense to both the patients and health professionals (Schipper *et al.*, 1990); and on the necessity for more formal assessments of quality of life in the context of clinical decision-making and day-to-day patient management. Establishment of quality of life parameters as valid and important outcome measures of health-care (Fallowfield,1990) has, in turn, led to widespread efforts to develop appropriate, meaningful and scientifically robust patient-based measures of quality of life. In the context of biomedicine and health care, the term 'quality of life' has generally been applied as the measurement of physical, social and psychological (as opposed to biochemical and physiological) function as perceived by the patient. While recognising that quality of life is influenced by many factors other than health (including income, job satisfaction, and social opportunities), health researchers have tended to focus on 'health-related quality of life', that is the perceived impact of health on an individual's physical, social and psychological well-being. Health-related quality of life (HRQOL) has been defined as 'the functional impact of an illness and its consequent therapy upon the patient as perceived by the patient' (Schipper *et al.*, 1986).

EPILEPSY AND HRQOL

The profound impact that epilepsy and seizures can have on the lives of those affected has been documented in many studies, both qualitative and quantitative. Areas highlighted as being of particular concern by people with epilepsy themselves include employment, driving, independence, lifestyle, mood, safety and cognitive problems (Fraser, 1980; Gilliam *et al.*, 1997; Fisher *et al.*, 2000). People with epilepsy have been shown to be at risk of reduced self-esteem and sense of self-worth, reduced sense of control, under- and un-employment (Fraser *et al.*, 1983; Collings, 1992), reduced rates of marriage and fertility (Dansky *et al.*, 1980; Lechtenberg, 1984; Sillanpää, 1992), social isolation and stigmatization (Jacoby, 1994; Baker *et al.*, 2000; Arnston *et al.*, 1986; Collings, 1992). People with epilepsy are more likely to experience and report a higher incidence of psychological problems (Ettinger *et al.*, 2004), physical comorbidities (Strine *et al.*, 2005), physical injuries (Buck *et al.*, 1997a) and neuropsychological problems (characterised as problems with attention, concentration and memory disorders) than are their peers without epilepsy. (Buck *et al.*, 1997a).

All these impacts are more commonly noted in people who develop chronic epilepsy, with seizures that prove intractable to treatment (Baker *et al.*, 1997), than in people whose seizures are well-controlled by antiepileptic medication, for whom epilepsy appears generally not to profoundly diminish the quality of their lives (Jacoby, 1992). Several studies have documented a clear linear relationship, for people with epilepsy, between seizure frequency and quality of life (Jacoby *et al.*, 1996; Baker *et al.*, 1997; Leidy *et al.*, 1999). However, it is also apparent from the work of several authors (Jacoby, 1992; Hermann, 1992; Baker *et al.*, 1997; Suurmeijer *et al.*, 2001) that the relationship between the severity of epilepsy and quality of life is complex and may be mediated by a number of different factors including: patients' own perceptions of themselves, the impact of their condition and its treatment; the influence of their family and interpersonal relationships; and general societal attitudes towards epilepsy.

A number of attempts have been made to understand the relationship between clinical and other non-clinical variables and HRQOL. For example, Baker and colleagues (1993) developed a three-level model to address operationally the impact of epilepsy and its treatment on patients' physical, social and psychological well-being. Wilson and Cleary (1995) advanced understanding of the possible inter-relationships between different variables by identifying factors influencing health outcome from biological markers through to overall HRQOL and the mediating role of psychological and emotional factors. Their model (see Figure 1) clearly highlights the complexity of these relationships in the face of chronic illness generally and epilepsy specifically. Work by Cramer and Spilker (1997) has highlighted how patient beliefs, values and judgements can act as a filter through which HRQOL outcomes of treatment can be influenced.

Figure 1.   Model adopted from Wilson & Clearly, 1995

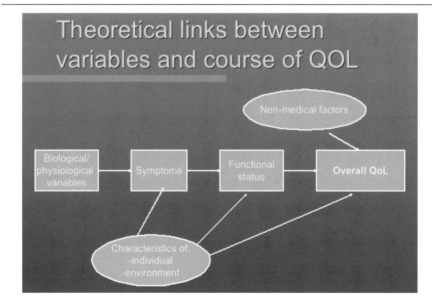

SEIZURE FREQUENCY AS AN OUTCOME MEASURE
IN PEOPLE WITH EPILEPSY

Traditionally, seizure frequency has been the commonest – and often the only – endpoint used in assessments of the efficacy of treatment for intractable epilepsy (Van Belle and Temkin, 1981). Trials designed to establish the efficacy of antiepileptic drugs have relied on time-to-first-seizure as the end point (Schofer and Temkin, 1986) or, in the case of double-blind crossover studies, a comparison of reduction of seizures during the active and placebo stages. The outcome is concluded as good for an antiepileptic drug trial where an individual patient achieves a greater than 50% reduction in seizure frequency without any serious adverse drug effects - even though most patients would agree that such a reduction, while worthwhile, is often not fully satisfactory (Schmidt, 1991). More recently, in trials outcome reporting, there has been a trend to report the number of patients rendered seizure-free or achieving a greater than 75% reduction.

Seizure frequency is also regarded as the principal measure of efficacy (Engel, 1987) in assessment of the outcome of surgery for patients with intractable epilepsy, success usually determined by the proportion of patients becoming seizure free (though recently attention has also been paid to HRQOL outcomes (Vickrey *et al.*, 1992)).

ROLE OF SEIZURE FREQUENCY FOR HRQOL

In one of the earliest studies focusing on the impact of frequent seizures on HRQOL, the authors (Thompson and Oxley, 1988) examined a group of patients with intractable epilepsy attending a specialist epilepsy assessment centre in the UK. Using the Social Problems Questionnaire, a measure assessing patient satisfaction with a number of key areas of daily functioning, they reported that almost a half of their respondents had received special schooling, only 11% were in employment, few were married and 57% reported not being in a stable relationship. A significant percentage (>70%) reported dissatisfaction with their social lives and their work situation, with a half reporting serious problems with their work situation and a third with their financial situation. Smith and colleagues (1991) in a later study using the same measure, reported somewhat lower levels of dissatisfaction among a group of patients with refractory epilepsy attending a hospital out-patient clinic. Baker and colleagues extended this research further by comparing patients with frequent seizures with those in remission and eligible for withdrawal of their antiepileptic drug medication (Baker *et al.*, 1996; Jacoby *et al.*, 1996). Operationalising QOL through a number of generic measures of perceived psychological well-being and health status, they demonstrated that patients with intractable epilepsy report higher levels of dysfunction in a number of different areas (see Table 1)

Table 1 Comparison of HRQOL measures for patients with intractable epilepsy v patients with epilepsy in remission

Measure	Patients with intractable epilepsy	Patients with epilepsy in remission
Self esteem	27.1	33.0
Mastery	18.1	21.7
NOTTINGHAM HEALTH PROFILE		
Energy	34	29
Pain	16	8
Emotional reaction	70	37
Sleep	41	28
Social isolation	51	15
Physical mobility	37	12

Jacoby and colleagues (1996) examined the role of seizure frequency in people with active epilepsy (which they defined as seizures or treatment for seizures in the previous two years) by comparing the HRQOL of patients who had experienced one or more seizures per month, less than one seizure per month or who had been seizure free in the last 12 months. Participants in the study were identified through 31 randomly selected general practioner practices in one health region in the UK (total practice population of 177,703; those with active epilepsy = 1341; prevalence rate of 0.8%; (Jacoby *et al.*, 1996; Baker *et al.*, 1996). There was a clear relationship between seizure activity and patients' perceptions of the impact of epilepsy and its treatment on their HRQOL. For example, patients with frequent seizures (>1 per month) were more than three times more likely to say that epilepsy and its treatment had a significant negative impact on their relationship with their family members, their social activities and their standard of living (see Figure 2).

Figure 2.   Comparison of percent (%) of patients reporting a significant impact score across the different domains

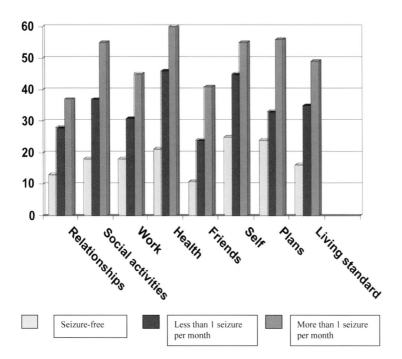

Leidy and colleagues also reported seizure frequency as an important determinant of HRQOL. HRQOL data obtained from 139 adults with epilepsy were compared with published norms for the US population; and the authors found that those who were seizure-free had similar HRQOL profiles to members of the general public without health problems; but that as seizure frequency increased, so patients reported increasingly impaired health status (Leidy *et al.*, 1999). These findings mirror those of Baker and colleagues (1997) for a large cohort of 5,000 people with epilepsy living in 15 countries in Europe. Respondents in this latter study were asked to provide a range of information, including details about their clinical status. In addition to questions relating directly to their experience of having epilepsy, respondents were also asked to complete a well-established generic health status measure, the Short-Form 36 (SF-36), for which UK population norms are available. The SF-36 includes 36 items addressing eight health concepts: physical functioning, social functioning, physical role limitations, emotional role limitations, mental health, energy/vitality, pain and general health. There were significant differences by seizure frequency in the way respondents scored for domains of the SF-36 (see Table 2).

Table 2.   Mean SF-36 scores by seizure frequency

| | Seizure frequency: | | |
Domain:	None in last year	Less than one A month	One or more a month	P-value
Physical functioning	88.9 (n=1948)	86.4 (n=1245)	79.2 (n=1942)	p<0.001
Social functioning	83.9 (n=1752)	76.1 (n=1140)	64.0 (n=1792)	p<0.001
Role limitations: physical	79.4 (n=1943)	70.7 (n=1237)	54.1 (n=1922)	p<0.001
Role limitations: emotional	77.7 (n=1933)	69.1 (n=1236)	59.0 (n=1917)	p<0.001
Mental health	70.0 (n=1940)	65.4 (n=1228)	61.2 (n=1913)	p<0.001
Energy/vitality	61.0 (n=1865)	55.8 (n=1168)	51.8 (n=1800)	p<0.001
Pain	74.0 (n=1939)	67.9 (n=1240)	59.2 (n=1915)	p<0.001
General health	69.7 (n=1893)	63.1 (n=1206)	58.0 (n=1824)	p<0.001

* Test of significance was Kruskal-Wallis one-way anova Baker *et al.*, 1997

The greatest differences were observed for limitations in emotional and physical functioning, but there were other domain differences that were likely also to be clinically significant. There were also differences by seizure frequency in the proportions reporting being stigmatised and reporting a marked impact of epilepsy on daily life and functioning, those with frequent seizures scoring positively for stigma and perceived impact more often than those with infrequent seizures or who were seizure-free (Baker *et al.*, 1997).

Most recently, Birbeck and colleagues (2002) compared changes in HRQOL across groups having different levels of change in seizure frequency (100%, 75-90%, 50-74% and 0-50%). They showed that those who became completely seizure-free (100%) experienced significantly more positive change on epilepsy-specific HRQOL measures than those continuing to have seizures. Based on their findings, they concluded that seizure reduction is insufficient to improve health-related quality of life and what is required is absolute seizure freedom.

SEIZURE FREQUENCY AND EPILEPSY SURGERY

Epilepsy surgery is now increasingly commonly considered an effective treatment for patients with intractable epilepsy, and there is accompanying recognition of the importance of patient-centred approaches to evaluating its success. A common finding in published studies of outcomes of surgery is that those patients rendered seizure-free report much better HRQOL outcomes than those with continuing seizures. Both retrospective and prospective studies have shown such improvements in surgery patients who either became completely seizure-free or whose seizures were dramatically reduced.

Langfitt (1995) demonstrated how seizure-freedom following surgery resulted in a significantly better HRQOL profile across a range of outcomes. This author studied three different groups of patients undergoing elective surgery for epilepsy: patients with complex partial seizures with secondary generalization; patients with complex partial seizures only; and a group of patients having undergone anterior temporal lobectomy and now seizure-free. The comparison demonstrated that those patients who were seizure-free reported better overall functioning than those with intractable partial seizures with or without secondarily generalization on three different outcome measures: the Washington Psychosocial Seizure Inventory (WPSI); the Epilepsy Surgery Inventory (ESI 55) and the Sickness Impact Profile (SIP). Interestingly, the most significant changes were seen on scores on the SIP (a generic measure) rather than the WPSI or ESI 55 (epilepsy specific measures).

Vickrey and colleagues (1994) examined HRQOL in 166 adults in the US who had undergone surgery for intractable epilepsy and found that after adjustment for age, gender, co-morbidity and level of education, the 55 completely seizure-free patients scored higher for HRQOL than patients with hypertension on the majority of SF-36 domains. The 67 patients still having seizures with impaired consciousness scored worse than those with hypertension or diabetic or heart disease patients. Malmgren and colleagues (1997) used the SF-36 to examine HRQOL in 103 epilepsy surgery patients in Sweden and reported a clear post-surgical HRQOL continuum, highest for patients rendered seizure-free without any aura, through to patients rendered seizure-free but with an aura, to those with a seizure reduction rate of 75-99% and, at the lowest end of the continuum, to patients in whom the seizure reduction rate was less than 75%.

These findings for the link between seizure freedom and quality of life are reiterated in studies by McLachlan and colleagues (1997) and Reid and colleagues (2004). These latter authors reported that in a longer term follow-up of epilepsy surgery patients (mean post-operative period 10.3 years), those patients who had remained seizure-free since surgery were more likely to have obtained employment, a driving license, and reported better psychological status, than those who had not (see Figure 3).

IMPACT OF SEIZURE AND
NON-SEIZURE RELATED FACTORS ON HRQOL

There is, then, a substantial body of evidence to support a direct link between seizure frequency and HRQOL. However, it is only with advances in statistical modelling techniques that the opportunity to study this relationship in detail has been made available. Jacoby and colleagues (1996), drawing evidence from a UK community study of epilepsy, examined the predictive

Figure 3. Psychosocial outcomes of surgery (Continuing seizures v Seizure-free)

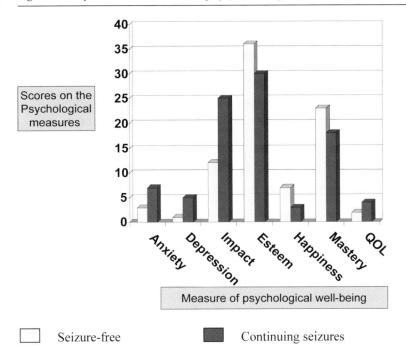

Seizure-free   Continuing seizures

value of seizure frequency on HRQOL outcomes in a group of people with active epilepsy (where active was defined as a history of seizures in the previous two years or seizure-free in that period, but on antiepileptic drugs) using multiple regression analysis. The authors were able to show that the frequency of seizures was the most significant predictor for a number of psychological and quality of life measures including: anxiety, depression, life fulfillment, perceived impact of epilepsy and self reported stigma – and this was true even when allowing for the role of clinical variables including age, sex, duration of epilepsy and age of onset. Similar findings were reported from a large cohort study by Baker and colleagues (1997) of the impact of epilepsy across a number of European countries.

However, factors other than seizure frequency are known to impact on patient perceived HRQOL. In the European study described above, seizure type was also shown to be indicative of quality of life, as measured by the SF-36 (Baker *et al.*, 1997), with patients experiencing multiple seizure types reporting poorest life quality. In a subsequent study involving 300 patients from France and Germany, seizure type and country of origin, as well as seizure frequency, were predictive of scores on a functional status question-naire (Baker *et al.*, 1998).

Smith and colleagues (1993) have suggested that seizure severity may be a more important determinant of psychosocial functioning than seizure frequency, particularly in patients with refractory epilepsy – though the relationship between seizure severity and HRQOL was found to be only modest in the study by Vickrey and colleagues (2000).   Patient perceived stigma has also been linked to HRQOL and psychosocial functioning (Baker *et al.*, 2000; Suurmeijer *et al.*, 2001). For example, in the study in Europe, high scores for stigma were correlated with worry, negative feelings about life and long-term health problems (Baker *et al.*, 2000). Furthermore, Dilorio and colleagues (2003) showed that patients with epilepsy who reported higher levels of stigma also reported lower levels of self-efficacy to manage their condition, more negative attitudes towards the possible outcomes of treatment and lower medication compliance, suggesting a possible circularity in the relationship between the different variables – stigma emerges as critical for QOL in people with epilepsy, both directly, in that perceived stigma impacts on psychosocial well-being; and indirectly, in that it impacts on treatment compliance and thus on seizure frequency or freedom.

Depression is the most common co-morbid condition associated with epilepsy and is present in 20-50% of persons with refractory epilepsy and 3-9% of persons with well-controlled epilepsy (Robertson, 1987).   Several studies have shown that depression is an important predictor of poor HRQOL. Lehrner and colleagues (1999) reported emotional impairment as a major problem in 56 people with temporal lobe epilepsy (TLE), with 45% of their sample scoring in the depressive range of a standard depression scale. Depression score was found to be a powerful predictor of self-reported quality of life after adjusting for seizure-related variables, demographic variables and cognitive functioning (IQ).   Though the small number of patients involved in the study limits the generalisabity of the findings, other studies have concluded similarly (Johnson *et al.*, 2004; Boylan *et al.*, 2004; Loring *et al.*, 2004).

Recently, there has been interest in how an individual's adjustment to their condition might influence their overall quality of life. Kemp and colleagues (1999) commented on the modest predictive power of clinical variables such as seizure frequency in predicting HRQOL in people with epilepsy and suggested that coping and illness representations might be of greater significance.   Utilising a novel measure of illness representations and a 'ways of coping' checklist, these authors reported that both contributed significantly to a positive emotional adjustment.   Goldstein and colleagues (2005) investigated the contribution of clinical variables including seizure frequency, coping strategies and illness representations to self-reported symptoms of anxiety and depression. These authors reported that the most significant predictors of anxiety and depression were 'escape avoidant' coping style scores. Once coping style had been taken into account, 'illness identity' scores (derived from an Illness Perception Questionnaire) accounted for a further significant amount of the variance for anxiety though not for depression.

The important question of how an individual's adjustment - or failure to adjust - to their condition affects their HRQOL has been the subject of research particularly in respect of the outcome of surgery for epilepsy. According to Wilson and colleagues (2004), patient and family expectations prior to treatment, and their willingness and ability, after treatment, to learn to discard roles associated with chronic illness, is crucial to a good outcome. The authors examined in detail patients' expectations of surgery and how this affected their perceptions of the success or failure of surgical intervention. Two major and distinct outcome subgroups could be identified: those who reported good outcomes, as characterised by improved family dynamics, enhanced vocational and social functioning, and driving by 24 months post-surgery; and those who reported poor outcomes, as characterised by affective disturbance at 12 months and difficulties discarding sick role behaviours (Wilson et al., 2005). These results clearly highlight the need to go beyond seizure frequency in understanding the impact of epilepsy and its treatment and the inadequacy of relying on seizure outcome as a means of determining the success or failure of treatment.

It has been proposed that a non-seizure frequency related means of improving quality of life would be increasing patients' knowledge of their condition, on the basis that increased knowledge results in increased compliance with treatment (Karoly, 1993), improved patient and physician communication (Baker et al., 1999), reductions in health risk behaviour (Helgeson et al., 1990) and improvements in psychological well-being (Jay et al., 1986). Certainly, it goes without saying that issues such as compliance are extremely important in the management of epilepsy and failure to comply is likely to have important negative impacts on the individual's life (Buck et al., 1997b; Cramer et al., 2004,). However, the evidence for increased knowledge having a direct and significant benefit on the quality of life of people with epilepsy remains limited.

Recently, the desire by people with epilepsy and their carers to be better informed about epilepsy has been highlighted (Baker, 2002). However, despite the increasing availability of information provided through epilepsy support groups, gaps in knowledge remain (Jain et al.,1993). In a European-wide study of over 6000 people with epilepsy, though levels of knowledge were generally acceptable, there was significant evidence that respondents lacked basic knowledge in respect of issues relating to medication and causes of epilepsy (Doughty et al., 2003). Importantly, given the focus of the present chapter, respondents with higher levels of knowledge were likely to report lower levels of stigma and lower levels of impact when compared to respondents with lower levels of knowledge (Doughty et al., 2003).

CONCLUSIONS

Many studies have demonstrated the commonly accepted dictum that the more severe the epilepsy, the worse the quality of life; and have emphasised that seizure freedom is an important pre-requisite for life quality. However, there are exceptions to the rule: not all people with well-controlled epilepsy report an enhanced quality of life and not all people with frequent seizures report a diminished one.   Rendering patients seizure-free must remain an important aim of treatment, but it cannot be assumed that to do so will de facto result in improvements to quality of life.   There is a clear body of evidence supporting that other factors including having to take medication, living with the fear of further seizures, being stigmatised and having difficulties adjusting to a diagnosis may exert a continuing negative impact. The challenge in the future will be to convert what we understand about the course, severity and impact of epilepsy into meaningful and manageable intervention strategies, which yield the best possible gains in terms of HRQOL improvements.

REFERENCES

Arnston, P., Drodge, D., Norton, R., Mundy, E. (1986). The perceived psychosocial consequences of having epilepsy. In: Whitman, S. and Hermann, B. (Eds) *Psychopathology in epilepsy: social dimensions*. Oxford University Press, Oxford. pp 143-166

Baker, G.A., Smith, D.F., Dewey, M. *et al.*, (1993). The initial development of a health-related quality of life model as an outcome measure in epilepsy. *Epilepsy Res* **16**, 65-81.

Baker, G.A., Gagnon, D. and McNulty, P. (1998). The relationships between seizure frequency, seizure type and quality of life: Findings from three European countries. *Epilepsy Res* **30**, 231-240.

Baker, G.A., Jacoby, A. and Chadwick, D.W. (1996). The associations of psychopathy and epilepsy: a community study. *Epilepsy res* **1**, 29-39.

Baker, G.A., Jacoby, A., Buck, D., Stalgis, C. and Monnet, D. (1997). Quality of life in people with epilepsy: a European study. *Epilepsia* **38**, 353-362.

Baker, G.A., Jacoby, A., DeBoer, H., Doughty, J., Myon, E. and Taieb, C. (1999). Patients' understanding of and adjustment to epilepsy: interim findings from a European survey. *Epilepsia* **40**, S26-29.

Baker, G.A., Brooks, J., Buck, D. and Jacoby, A. (2000). The stigma of epilepsy: a European perspective *Epilepsia* **41**, 98-104.

Baker, G.A. (2002). People with epilepsy: what do they know and understand, and how does this contribute to their perceived level of stigma? *Epilepsy Behav* **3**, 26-32.

Birbeck, G.L., Hays, R.D., Cui, X. and Vickrey, B.G. (2002). Seizure reduction and quality of life improvements in people with epilepsy. *Epilepsia* **43**, 535-538.

Boylan, L.S., Flint, L.A., Labovitz, D.L., Jackson, S.C., Starner, K. and Devinsky, O. (2004). Depression but not seizure frequency predicts quality of life in treatment-resistant epilepsy. *Neurology* **62**, 258-261.

Buck, D., Baker, G.A., Smith, D.F., Jacoby, A., Graham-Jones, S. and Chadwick, D.W. (1997a). Patients experience of epilepsy as a result of epilepsy. *Epilepsia* **38**, 439-444.

Buck, D., Jacoby, A., Baker, G.A. and Chadwick, D.W. (1997b). Factors influencing compliance with antiepileptic drug regimes. *Seizure* **6**, 87-93.

Collings, J. (1990). Psychosocial well being and epilepsy: an empirical study. *Epilepsia* **31**, 418-426.

Collings, J. (1992). *Epilepsy and the experience of employment. A report of a national survey by the British Epilepsy Association.* British Epilepsy Association. Leeds.

Cramer, J.A. and Spilker, B, (1997). *Quality of Life Pharmacoeconomics: An Intoduction*. Lippincott Williams.

Cramer, J.A., Hammer, A.E. and Kustra, R. (2004). Quality of life improvement with conversion to lamotrigine monotherapy. *Epilepsy Behav* **5**, 224-230.

Dansky, L.V., Andermann, E. and Andermann, F. (1980). Marriage and fertility in epileptic patients. *Epilepsia* **21**, 261-271.

Dilorio, C., Shafer, P.O., Letz, R., Henry, T., Schomer, D.L. and Yeager, K. (2003). The association of stigma with self-management and perceptions of health care among adults with epilepsy. *Epilepsy Behav* **4**, 259-267.

Doughty, J., Baker, G.A., Jacoby, A. and Lavaud, V. (2003) Cross-cultural differences in levels of knowledge about epilepsy. *Epilepsia*. **44**, 115-123.

Engel, J. (1987). *Surgical treatment of the epilepsies*. Raven Press, New York.

Ettinger, A., Reed, M. and Cramer, J. (2004). Depression and comorbidity in community-based patients with epilepsy or asthma. *Neurology* **63**, 1008-1014.

Fallowfield, L. (1990). *The quality of life: The missing measurement in health care.* Souvenir Press. London, England.

Fisher, R.S., Vickrey, B.G., Gibson, P,, Hermann, B., Penovich, P. and Scherer, A. and Walker S (2000). The impact of epilepsy from the patient's perspective: description and subjective perceptions. *Epilepsy Res* **41**, 39-51.

Fraser, R. (1980). Vocational aspects of epilepsy. In: Hermann, B (Ed), *A multidisciplincary handbook of epilepsy.* Springfield, Illinois.

Fraser, R.T., Clemmons, D., Trjo, W. and Temkin, N.R. (1983). Program evaluation in epilepsy rehabilitation. *Epilepsia* **24**, 734-746.

Gilliam, F., Kuzniecky, R., Faught, E., Black, L., Carpenter, G. and Schrodt, R. (1997). Patient-validated content of epilepsy-specific QOL measurement. *Epilepsia* **38**, 233-236.

Goldstein, L.H., Holland, L., Soteriou, H. and Mellers, J.D. (2005). Illness representations, coping styles and mood in adults with epilepsy. *Epilepsy Res* **67**, 1-11.

Helgeson, D.C., Mittan, R., Tan, S.Y. and Charyasirisobhon, S. (1990). Sepulveda Epilepsy Education: the efficacy of a psychoeducational treatment program in treating medical and psychosocial aspects of epilepsy. *Epilepsia* **31**, 75-82.

Hermann, B.P. (1992). Quality of life in epilepsy. *J Epilepsy* **5**, 153-165.

Jacoby, A. (1992). Epilepsy and the quality of everyday life. Findings from a study of well-controlled epilepsy. *Soc Sci Med* **34**, 657-666.

Jacoby, A. (1994). Felt versus enacted stigma: a concept revised. *Soc Sci Med* **38**, 269-274.

Jacoby, A., Baker, G.A., Steen, N., Potts, P. and Chadwick, D.W. (1996). The clinical course of epilepsy and its psychosocial correlates: findings from a U.K. Community study. *Epilepsia* **37**,148-161.

Jain, P., Patterson, V.H. and Morrow, J.I. (1993). What people with epilepsy want from a hospital clinic. *Seizure* **2**, 75-78.

Jay, S., Elliott, C. and Varni, J.W. (1986). Acute and chronic pain in adults and children with cancer. *J Consult Clin Psychol* **54**, 601-607.

Johnson, E.K., Jones, J.E., Seidenberg, M. and Hermann, B.P. (2004). The relative impact of anxiety, depression and clinical seizure features on health-related quality of life in epilepsy. *Epilepsia* **45**, 544-550.

Karoly, P. (1993). Enlarging the scope of the compliance construct: Toward developmental and motivational relevance. In: Epstein, L.H. *et al.*, (Ed), *Developmental aspects of health compliance behaviour.*: Lawrence Erlbaum Associates. Hillsdale, NJ; England. pp11-27.

Kemp, S., Morley, S. and Anderson, E. (1999). Coping with epilepsy: Do illness representations play a role? *Brit J Clin Psychol* **38**, 43-58.

Langfitt, J.T. (1995). Comparison of the psychometric characteristics of three quality of life measures in intractable epilepsy. *Qual Life Res* **4**, 101-114.

Lechtenberg, R. (1984). *Epilepsy and the family.* Harvard University Press. Cambridge, MA.

Lehrner, J., Kalchmayr, R., Serles, W., Olbrich, A., Pataraia, E., Aull, S., Bacher, J., Leutmezer, F., Groppel, G., Deecke, L. and Baumgartner, C. (1999). Health-related quality of life (HRQOL), activity of daily living (ADL) and depressive mood disorder in temporal lobe epilepsy patients. *Seizure* **8**, 88-92.

Leidy, N.K., Elixhauser, A., Vickrey, B., Means, E. and Willian, M.K. (1999). Seizure frequency and health-related quality of life of adults with epilepsy. *Neurology* **53**, 162-166.

Loring, D., Meador, K.J. and Lee, G.P. (2004). Determinants of quality of life in epilepsy. *Epilepsy Behav* **5**, 976-980.

Malmgren, K., Sullivan, M., Ekstedt, G., Kullsberg, G. and Kumlien, E. (1997). Health-related quality of life after epilepsy surgery: a Swedish multicentre study. *Epilepsia* **38**, 830-838.

McLachlan, R.S., Rose, K.J., Derry, P., Bonnar, C., Blume, W.T., Girvin, J.P. (1997). Health related quality of life and seiure control in temporal lobe epilepsy. *Ann Neurol* **41**, 482-489.

Reid, K., Herbert, A. and Baker, G.A. (2004). Epilepsy surgery: patient perceived long-term costs and benefits. *Epilepsy Behav* **5**, 81-87.

Robertson, M.M. (1987). Depression in patients with epilepsy reconsidered. In: Pedley, T.A. and Meldrum, B.S. (Eds), *Recent advances in epilepsy 4*. Churchill Livingstone, Edinburgh, London, Melbourne, New York. pp 205-240.

Schipper, H., Clinch, J. and Powell, V. (1990). Definitions and conceptual issues. In: Spilker, B. (Ed), *Quality of Life Assessment in Clinical Trials*. Raven Press, NY. pp 11-24.

Schipper, H., Clinch, J., McMurray, A.and Levitt, M. (1986). Measuring the quality of life of cancer patients: the Functional Living Index for Cancer: development and validation. *J Clin Oncol* **2**, 472-483.

Schmidt, D. (1991). Evaluation of clinical efficacy in antiepileptic drug trials. *Epilepsy Res Supp* **3**, 69-77.

Schofer, J.B. and Temkin, N.R. (1986). Comparison of alternative outcome measures for antiepileptic drug trials. *Arch Neurol* **43**, 877-881.

Sillanpää, M. (1992). Epilepsy in children: Prevalence, disability and handicap. *Epilepsia* **33**, 444-449.

Smith, D.F., Baker, G.A., Davies, G., Dewey, M. and Chadwick, D.W. (1991). Randomized, placebo-controlled, double-blind crossover trial of lamotrigine as add-on therapy in patients with refractory epilepsy. *Epilepsia* **32**, 51.

Smith, D.F., Baker, G.A., Jacoby, A., Chadwick, D.W. (1993). The contribution of the measurement of seizure severity to quality of life research. *Quality of Life Research: An International Journal of Quality of Life Aspects of Treatment, Care and Rehabilitation*. **4**, 143-158.

Strine, T.W., Kobau, R., Chapman, D.P., Thurman, D.J., Price, P. and Balluz, L.S. (2005). Psychological distress, comorbidities and health behaviours among US adults with seizures: results from the 2002 National Health Interview Survey. *Epilepsia* **46**, 1133-1139.

Suurmeijer, T.P.B.M., Reuvekamp, M.F. and Aldenkamp, B.P. (2001). Social functioning, psychological functioning and quality of life in epilepsy. *Epilepsia* **42**, 1160-1168.

Thompson, P.J. and Oxley, J. (1988). Socioeconomic accompaniments of severe epilepsy. *Epilepsia* **29 (Suppl 1)**, S9-S18.

Van Belle, G. and Temkin, N. (1981). Design strategies in the clinical evaluation of new antiepileptic drugs. In: Pedley, T.A. and Meldrum, B.S. (Eds), *Recent Advances in Epilepsy*. Church & Livingstone. London, Melboure, New York. pp 93-111.

Vickrey, B.G., Berg, A.T., Sperling, M.R., Shinnar, S., Langfitt, J.T. *et al.* (2000). Relationships between seizure severity and health-related quality of life in refractory localisation-related epilepsy. *Epilepsia* **41**, 760-764.

Vickrey, B.G., Hays, R.D., Graber, R.J. and Rausch, R. (1992). A health-related quality of life instrument for patients evaluate for epilepsy surgery. *Medical Care* **30**, 299-319.

Vickrey, B.G., Hays, R.D., Rausch, R., Sutherling, W.W., Engel, J. Jr. and Brook, R.H. (1994). Quality of life of epilepsy surgery patients as compared with outpatients with hypertension, diabetes, heart disease and/or depressive symptoms. *Epilepsia* **35**, 597-607.

Wilson, B. and Cleary, P.D. (1995). Linking clinical variables with health-related quality of life: A conceptual model of patient outcomes. *JAMA* **273**, 59-65.

Wilson, S.J., Bladin, P.F. and Saling, M.M. (2004). Paradoxical results in the cure of chronic illness: the "burden of normality" as exemplified following seizure surgery. *Epilepsy Behav* **5**, 13-21.

Wilson, S.J., Bladin, P.F., Saling, M.M. and Pattison, P.E. (2005). Characterizing psychosocial outcome trajectories following seizure surgery *Epilepsy Behav* **6**, 570-580.

Index

Page numbers in *italics* refer to figures and tables.